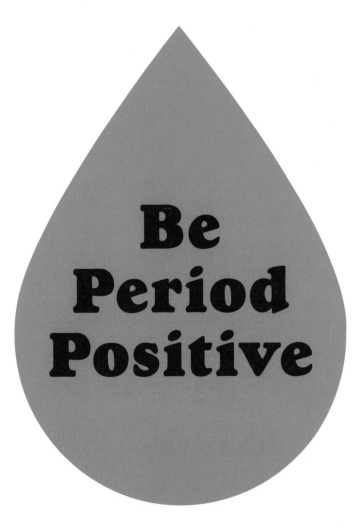

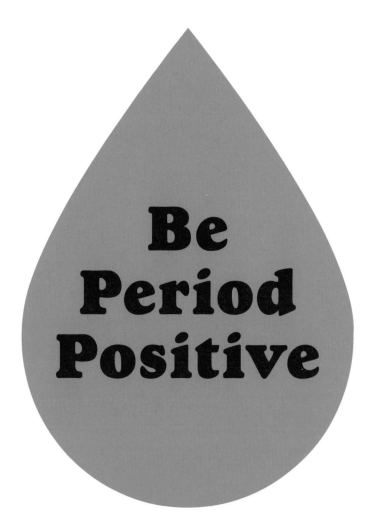

Be Period Positive

Reframe your thinking and reshape
the future of menstruation

CHELLA QUINT

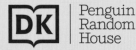

Editor Megan Lea
US Editor Kayla Dugger
US Executive Editor Lori Cates Hand
Designer Natalie Clay
Design Assistant Vanessa Hamilton
Senior Editors Salima Hirani, Emma Hill
Project Art Editor Louise Brigenshaw
Jacket Designer Amy Cox
Jacket Coordinator Lucy Philpott
Pre-production Producer David Almond
Producer Luca Bazzoli
Creative Technical Support Sonia Charbonnier
Managing Editor Dawn Henderson
Managing Art Editor Marianne Markham
Art Director Maxine Pedliham
Publishing Director Katie Cowan

Medical Consultant Shehnaaz Jivraj
Illustrator Céleste Wallaert

First American Edition, 2021
Published in the United States by DK Publishing
1450 Broadway, Suite 801, New York, NY 10018

Copyright © 2021 Dorling Kindersley Limited
DK, a Division of Penguin Random House LLC
21 22 23 24 25 10 9 8 7 6 5 4 3 2 1
001–322895–Jul/2021

Printed and bound in China

The Period Positive logo, and STAINS™ are
registered trademarks and are used with
permission from Chella Quint.

For more information go to:
www.periodpositive.com

For the curious
www.dk.com

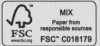

This book was made with Forest Stewardship Council™
certified paper—one small step in DK's commitment to
a sustainable future.
For more information go to www.dk.com/our-green-pledge

Contents

Hello! I'm so glad you're here!

By the end of this book, you will have the tools you need to reclaim menstruation. It took me a long time to build this toolkit, but I wrote *Be Period Positive* so it doesn't take you as long as it took me to feel better about periods! It's written Q&A style, because not being afraid to ask questions is essential to being period positive.

Growing up, I had *tons* of questions about periods, but I never knew who'd be comfortable answering them. Maybe it was like that for you, too? I wished for older siblings, for superheroes, even for someone on TV to at least talk about periods without them being seen as a secret or as the butt of the joke.

And periods certainly weren't a laughing matter for me back then. The same year mine started, I had a *major* leaking incident at the very first slumber party I ever attended. I was 12 and a half, and—I kid you not—it was during a *huge blizzard*, so we were snowed in and my parents couldn't come get me. That night, I experienced the full mortification that period leaks can cause, including the onslaught of major teasing that followed from other kids socialized to feel as ashamed of periods as I

was. Back then, I imagined a superhero named Over Flo and wished she would come and save the day. But believing that a leak should equal public humiliation is evidence that we've internalized the messages we've received about periods. This doesn't have to represent the relationship we have with our bodies. It took *years* before I was ready to think about that night again. When I finally did, I asked myself, *What if I became my own superhero ... with the power to challenge ads and embrace stains?* I created a zine called *Adventures in Menstruating*, and this was the first story I told. I began rejecting the shaming advertising messages that I saw around me and reimagined period stains as a high-end fashion emblem, turning it into a comedy art installation. (I named it STAINS™, and you'll see this parody brand throughout the book!)

As I got older, my friends and audiences and I wanted to know more: about hormones and contraception and fertility and what menopause would be like. Asking questions is brave in the face of taboo. I wanted everyone to be confident enough to ask about periods, and clued in enough to share the answers with others. I found that using humor was the best way to break the ice when people felt uncomfortable and that joy was the best antidote to shame. The zine became a touring comedy show, and I gave workshops to schools and colleges while teaching middle and high school health education and studying for a Master's in menstruation education. Through interactions with audiences and workshop attendees, I tried to pin down what it was starting to mean to be period positive. At first, I focused on general things: talking about menstruation out loud, including everyone in the conversation, not being afraid to ask questions, knowing how to chart a cycle, and challenging messages about blood and leaking.

Then I started to get specific. I tested a curriculum model. I imagined what period positive schools and workplaces and cities would be and designed the Period Positive award logo. I developed the Period Positive Pledge to encourage others to create campaigns that were both challenging and inclusive. I shared these ideas with different communities and other artists, and eventually with large organizations and governments,

close to home and around the world. That grew into Period Positive Global Champions: a growing network of like-minded activists and researchers learning from each other and developing best practices together.

And all of those key moments for me started by asking questions. I hope that picking up this book becomes a key moment for you in challenging menstrual taboos and that it empowers you to ensure that you get the answers you need from doctors, corporations, partners, bosses, teachers, and politicians.

This book came directly from real questions asked by real menstruators. That doesn't mean you shouldn't read this if you don't menstruate—I hope the information in these pages is helpful for anyone navigating these topics. Seeing individuals turn their attitudes around and feel better about periods is so heartening. It motivates me to continue to invite others to help make the world a more period positive place, and that's why this book is for you.

Chella x

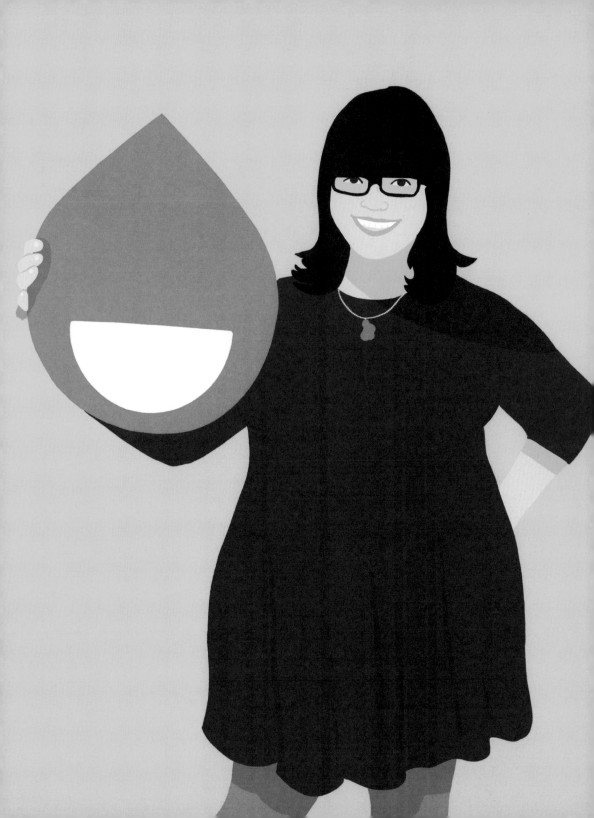

"Be period positive" is an invitation.

A lot of us carry around shame and discomfort about our bodies. Social stigmas around bodily functions and sexual health can be a real driver of embodied shame. Periods and menstrual taboos can affect our well-being so much more than we realize.

At the heart of it, period positivity is a three-part idea:

1. The way we talk, think, and feel about periods does not have to be negative, even if—especially if—our experience with menstruation has been less than positive. You don't have to love periods, but there is so much value in talking about them.

2. We can actively do things to change how we frame menstruation—as individuals, in the media, and in society—and this will help us feel happier and healthier and make more informed decisions.

3. Being inclusive and sharing this approach will help more and more people try out this mindset, leading to a transformation of the whole topic in our global culture.

It's totally possible—we've done it before! Unfortunately, most communities in the world have not held onto the good relationships we've had with periods on and off throughout history, and it's been particularly noticeable over the last century or so. Many people have internalized the idea that periods should be secret or hidden, and it's hard to break out of that thought pattern. Being period positive is a liberating, mindful way to challenge this within ourselves and address it with others. You'd be surprised how many other seemingly unrelated issues fall into place once you feel better about periods—whether you have them or not!

In my work on Period Positive, I realized the best way to create transformative change that could be relevant anywhere was to develop a framework that anyone could use to ensure that when they talked about period positivity, they were being community minded, inclusive, and intersectional. I want the Period Positive Pledge to become a blueprint that will encourage people to not just question the status quo, but work to ensure that menstrual activism, advocacy, and policy put people before profit and include all genders.

Let's get started

I started this project in 2005; coined the phrase "period positive" in 2006; and have been doing activism, education, and research ever since, picking up more and more colleagues and friends along the way. Things have improved since then, but there's a way to go, and a lot of us have met with the same issue—we're still surrounded by taboos. That's down to how much our view of menstruation has been affected by historic corporate media messages and their influence on how we learned about

EVERY INDIVIDUAL HAS THE
POWER
TO CHALLENGE MENSTRUAL TABOOS

periods. Words like "secret," "whisper," and "discreet"; a fear of leaks; the habit of hiding menstrual products; and a focus on concealing periods keep us in "period panic mode." As we start to influence government policy, better education and media literacy must become our essential foundations. This will enable us to reject embodied shame and truly understand how the issues all fit together. Then we can develop the best possible plans to address the

health and financial inequalities around menstruation and reproductive justice. It starts with asking questions, and I hope this book will help you answer yours.

Chapter 1, **History**, is a bit of a period drama—we'll look at periods of the past and debunk misinformation. Chapter 2 is a deep dive into **Period positivity**—how to start shifting your mindset and developing new ways of looking at places, people, and practices within the menstrual discourse. Chapter 3 explores all things **Blood**—what menstrual blood is, why it happens, how to talk about it, and how to manage it. Chapter 4 covers the wide world of **Hormones**—how the chemicals that travel around our bodies set the whole process in motion every cycle, keep it going, and influence different aspects of our reproductive health. In Chapter 5, you'll find all the information you need to understand the ins and outs and ups and downs of **Fertility and contraception**, and Chapter 6 gives us reasons to be cheerful about the next phase of life, busting the many, many myths surrounding **Perimenopause and menopause**.

Becoming period positive is way easier than you think. Keep on reading—it's going to be an awesome adventure!

"Building our relationship
with periods and
reproductive health
is powerful and necessary."

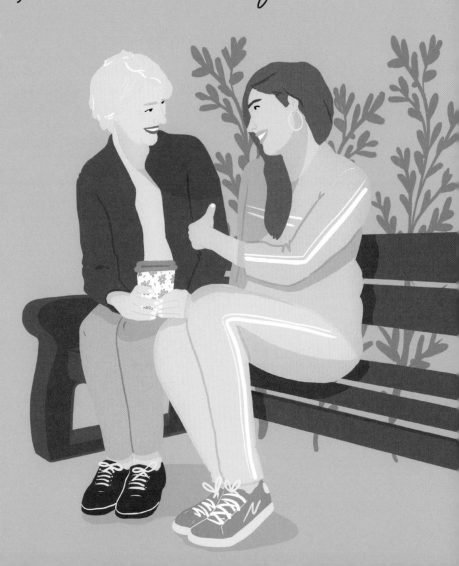

History

Let's start at the very beginning—or, at least as far back as we can reliably go. In order to understand exactly why all things period are seen and talked about as they are now, we need to time travel a little bit. Get ready to bust myths, dig around for any grains of truth in some wild superstitions, and pin down how today's taboos gained such problematic staying power.

Why do we have periods?

That's a really good question! To answer it, we need to think of ourselves as a species. We do what every other animal does—reproduce. Periods are just a part of how our species does it.

A period, or menstruation, is the result of ovulation—which seems to be the less famous half of the menstrual cycle. Humans ovulate regularly (see page 86) to improve our chances of reproducing, and the womb grows a lining to help this along. If the egg is fertilized and conception happens, the lining stays in place throughout the pregnancy, enabling the placenta to embed itself in it as it grows, so it can provide nutrients to the developing fetus. The uterine lining is pretty important. No uterine lining, no placenta, no fetus, no more humans—so it's pretty essential for us that this all happens. If the egg remains unfertilized, though, our bodies no longer need the lining, and we bleed. And then the cycle begins again. For us, menstrual cycles happen every 21–35 days. (See page 89 for more on cycle length.)

Menstruating animals

Some primates menstruate, along with some species of bats and rodents, including the elephant shrew.

Frequency

You could say that "little and often" is how we are fertile, while other animals are less frequently fertile, but in a more controlled way—in response to mating triggers. There are evolutionary pluses and minuses either way. On the bright side, humans don't usually have to do anything special to trigger fertility—it just happens. On the downside, we have to actively interrupt the cycle if we don't want to make any humans that month, or ever. Swings and roundabouts. It could be different. We could be reptiles or birds or platypuses, and lay eggs. Or reproduce through parthenogenesis. Or clone ourselves. (Did I just make it weird?)

Now, if, instead of the evolutionary history of menstruating, what you were *really* wondering about was "Why oh why are we so unlucky as to have periods?", the answer is … "Unlucky? But periods are actually amazing!" And in the following 99 questions and answers, I will do my best to expand on that, so that by the end of this book, you will be the most confident, comfortable, and knowledgeable menstruator in the land!

SEXUAL REPRODUCTION ENABLES GENETIC VARIATION SO EACH GENERATION CAN ADAPT TO NEW ENVIRONMENTS, IMPROVING SURVIVAL

What were periods like in the past?

People have been bleeding since prehistoric times, but little of that is written down, so we rely on speculation to paint a picture of a lost history of menstruation.

Some speculation is based on chemical analysis of digestion, bone structure, and minerals in teeth, while some is inspired by written historical accounts. Anthropologists and historians have interpreted clues, but some of these interpretations are subjective and often conflicting. By the time history was being recorded, we'd been menstruating for millennia, and the people doing the chiseling, writing, scribing, and illuminating at the time were mostly people who didn't get periods. So what we "know" isn't a whole lot until we start focusing on the insights of much more recent research.

Celestial reference

In Neolithic times, we can guess that, due to sparser nutrition, considerable physical exertion, and nomadic lifestyles, people may have begun menstruating at a later age than they do today. But without actual evidence, we can't confirm this.

We do know that, for ancient people, using calendars and mapping celestial bodies was essential for agriculture and navigation and that calendars evolved from tracking the sun, moon, planets, and stars. The Latin word for

"months" is *menses*, which was first recorded as being used to mean "menstrual flow" in the late 15th century. So we can extrapolate that menstrual flow occurred monthly-ish back in the 1500s, as it does today.

Also, historians have noted (from primary sources like letters) that in the Early Modern period (around 1500–1815), periods started between the ages of 12–14 (similar to today) and ended around age 49 (just a little earlier than they do today). Because life expectancy was shorter, fewer people lived as long past menopause as they do now. (See pages 140–153 for more on menopause.)

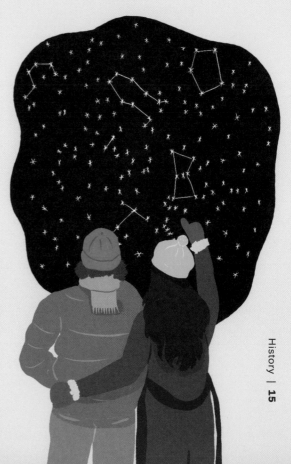

What did our ancestors believe about menstruation?

It's difficult to know how people might have felt about periods in ancient times, as menstruation has been shrouded in taboos, but there are echoes in historical sources that give us some clues.

Ancient cultures associated menstruation with power due to its link with creating life, and blood was seen as an essential life force. But this power was interpreted both negatively and positively, even within the same cultures.

A link between menstruation and purity can also be traced to ancient religions, and different interpretations of purity can color how that's reflected in modern analysis. The power of fertility was seen as a highly concentrated or pure power. This concept, it is believed, led to seclusion during the sacred process of menses, which was often embraced by menstruators, to acknowledge the sacredness with separation. The influence of patriarchal attitudes distorted this concept in many cases, so that controlling restrictions were often used to stop menstruators practicing certain activities.

Menstruation in science

Ancient Greek and Roman doctors were highly influential. Throughout the last two millennia, modern practitioners, even when they disagreed, still followed their teachings.

Some of those misguided beliefs have been emulated over the past 2,000 years – a few right up until the last century. For example, from ancient times to only a couple of centuries ago, many doctors held that menstruation naturally balanced the "four humors" that were believed to make up the body and used bloodletting to mimic this process as a treatment for various illnesses. In 2 CE, physicians of the Roman Empire couldn't agree on whether the uterus had its own sense of smell or could move around the entire body at will, but that didn't stop a 17th-century British doctor from writing about his theory of the "wandering womb" causing sickness wherever it went.

"HYSTERIA"—
FROM THE LATIN FOR UTERUS—WAS SAID TO BE CAUSED BY THE **UTERUS WANDERING THE BODY**. THE TERM IS NO LONGER CLINICALLY RECOGNIZED.

In Rome two millennia ago, the philosopher Pliny the Elder wrote that one touch from a menstruating woman could kill crops, fog a mirror, turn wine to vinegar, blunt a sword, or rust metal! You may laugh, but in the early 20th century, it was believed that there were poisonous "menotoxins" in menstrual blood. Persistent superstitions fed into modern ideas of periods being dirty (see pages 26–27). Some believed them, but despite the taboos, many people were amused by them, and on and off, there have been times throughout history when people have talked freely about menstruation.

Do any societies celebrate people on their period?

In many cultures and faiths, a rite of passage, ritual, or ceremony exists to mark the start of periods or a general coming of age, but the word "celebrate" is subjective when it comes to attitudes to menstruation.

First period ceremonies

Sometimes parents acknowledging their child growing up is a rite of passage in name only. For other families, this may be a nice excuse for a large celebration. Young people may find the attention exposing, or embrace it. They may wish to keep their bodily functions private, or simply see the communal sharing of this information as safe and natural. The more supportive versions of these practices focus on older menstruators in the family bestowing symbols of maturity, sharing nutrient-rich foods, and imparting practical advice about periods and puberty. However, when these celebrations are linked to fertility and coming of age, there may be added expectations around sex, relationships, and marriage that can cause the young person to feel fearful and anxious.

Cycle rituals

As with first period (or menarche) events, menstrual rituals that transmit positive and empowering activities often co-exist alongside versions that became connected to patriarchal control or messages that menstrual blood is dirty or impure. Some menstruators embrace the very same rituals and practices as celebratory that their friends and neighbors have questioned or rejected. They may value private time with other menstruators and appreciate time to rest.

Reclaim and reconstruct

The most valued and valuable practices seem to be co-created celebrations where *everyone* consents to the practice and values it. In recent years, people have begun to throw first-period parties for their friends, their kids, and themselves. Some of these celebrations may be tongue-in-cheek, pun-filled extravaganzas, with red velvet cake and shark piñatas, while others are more earnest and spiritual affairs. Both kinds aim to reclaim or reimagine a part of our cultural history that celebrates periods as something healthy and positive.

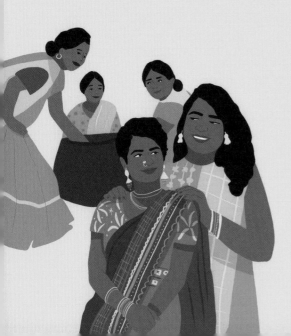

Celebrating menarche
In parts of India, a girl is gifted her first half-sari in the Ritu Kala Samskara ceremony.

How did people manage menstruation in history?

Before the advent of modern menstrual products, people often relied on scraps of fabric to absorb period blood. Many early cultures recorded the materials used for this purpose.

Collecting sphagnum moss, a naturally absorbent plant, must have been something many of our ancestors did, as it was a popular first aid material around the world. In several places, there are specific examples of it being used as a menstrual product before bandages were widely available (see opposite). Ancient Egyptians, Greeks, and Romans used sphagnum moss to manage periods and made folded pads of papyrus, flax, wool, and woven fabrics.

Across the globe, pieces of clean, folded fabric, referred to in Early Modern Britain as clouts or rags (hence the euphemism "on the rag"), were widely used to protect clothing.

Inspiration from nature
Sphagnum moss was used to absorb blood before bandages were in common use.

In medieval Europe, periods were considered unclean and were often hidden but were less taboo by the Early Modern era, with primary sources giving us some insight into the logistics of menstrual management at the time.

Red petticoats
This may surprise you, but in Early Modern and Victorian times, free bleeding (not using menstrual products) was common in the British working classes. In Victorian factories, sawdust was spread on the floor to absorb the blood of menstruating workers. At the end of the day, the sawdust was swept away and replaced. According to the accounts of workers and industrialists, people talked about their periods, and it was considered a normal part of the working day to accommodate menstruating staff. People also used extra layers of clothing to catch their menstrual blood and often had a specific set of petticoats or aprons made from absorbent fabric, or sometimes rubber, to keep the more expensive outer layers of their clothing clean and free of stains.

How did commercial menstrual products develop?

At the start of the 20th century, people still used homemade products. By mid-century, disposable commercial products had become ubiquitous. But things are changing!

During World War I, nurses used spare bandages to manage their periods. After the war, bandage manufacturers rebranded surplus supplies as disposable menstrual products. These early pads were sold on a strip and cut from the roll. They evolved into pads in a box that people pinned into their underwear.

Tampons were developed in the 1930s but only caught on around mid-century. Likewise, menstrual cups, originally made of rubber, were first advertised in the 1930s.

From the 1970s onward, designers developed contoured pads, added adhesive backing, and brought in new shapes and lengths. Incorporating synthetic ingredients led to thinner pads with higher absorbency and individual wrappers. The most recent innovation was wings to help pads stay in place and prevent blood from leaking over the sides.

In the early 21st century, silicone menstrual cups and cloth pads resurged, their comfort and sustainability now making them popular alternatives. Most recently, period underwear has been a big hit. Although disposable products have reached all parts of the globe, many people still use, or have returned to using, fabric to absorb their blood.

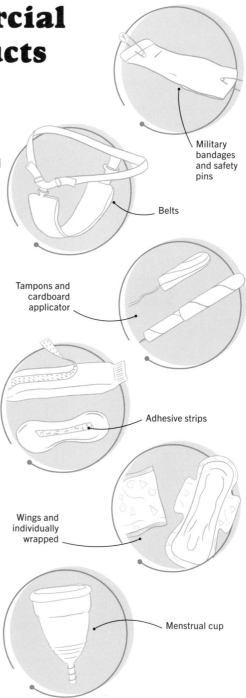

Military bandages and safety pins

Belts

Tampons and cardboard applicator

Adhesive strips

Wings and individually wrapped

Menstrual cup

Why is the advertising of commercial menstrual products significant?

Over the years, advertising messages have had (and still do have) a hugely negative influence on our attitudes to periods. It's highly freeing to understand how and why these messages work.

People had age-old routines for managing periods when commercial menstrual products were invented in the 1920s and 30s (see page 19), so it was going to be a tough sell. Advertisers had to go big or go home—and wow, did they go big! They did so by focusing on menstruation-related fears and embarrassment in order to sell products to relieve those same invented negative feelings. This revived old myths around dirt and fear and set the tone for a global industry. We still feel the reverberations of those early hard-sell messages in ads and other menstrual media today. The ads may have originated in North America, but the companies—and their messages—were soon multinational.

1920s—A hygiene nightmare!
The earliest ads from the 1920s were often framed as letters from doctors and established a link between periods and ideas of hygiene and embarrassment. One ad from 1926 was headed with the words "A Great Hygienic Handicap that Your Daughter will be Spared." It claimed that, without the product, people would experience fear and terror and that "80% of women in the better walks of life" were their customers, positioning the product as an aspirational brand. It explained how the "sanitary" pad advertised would solve "woman's oldest hygienic problem," "the most trying of hygienic conditions," and assured would-be consumers that it was nonvisible through clothing. It was sold "ready-wrapped in plain paper" to "save embarrassment."

The clear messages, still present in ads today, were that periods are unhygienic, embarrassing, to be hidden, and that classy people use the latest "scientific" products rather than DIY versions. And it just went on from there.

1930s—Aggghhhh, leaks!!
In 1935, another North American product was advertised in newspapers and magazines with the header "Women! End accident-panic!", showing a picture of a woman who looked as

Missed USP
The unique selling point of disposable menstrual products was their obvious convenience, yet advertisers chose to focus on fear.

though she were watching a horror movie. Like others of the era, this ad focused on leakage horror, promising to end the panic by offering "complete protection from embarrassing 'accidents.'" But there hadn't really been any panic in the past—leaks were just ... managed. These ad campaigns, with their emotive language and images, invented the fear of leaks and stains so people would pay to be protected from the "haunting fear of accidents" that they were told they had! If you think about it, this fear still impacts many decisions we make about menstrual products, clothes we wear, places we go ... And in ads today, leaks remain the enemy.

1940s—Shhhhh!

Speaking of enemies, during the 1940s, ads took on a wartime feel, with words like "shield," "safety," and "protection" coming into play. The concept of whispering in an era of wartime secrets also became common. The message was that if you *had* to talk about your period, you shouldn't do so out loud.

The industry is still known as "sanitary protection," and the words "whisper," "secret," and "discreet" are ubiquitous. In fact, some companies brag about their wrappers being so silent that no one in the next cubicle can hear you unwrap one. This type of messaging encourages people to hide their periods—even from other menstruators.

Shameful secret
Advertising often described or depicted whispering, tacitly imploring customers to stay silent.

1950s—Periods? What periods?

Things got even more sanitized in the 1950s. Now the message was "Don't let people see your products!" One ad promised that their boxes of pads were disguised so well that when a "housewife" was asked what she thought they contained, she replied, "It's bath salts! No, it's candy!" This ad proudly promoted products for hiding your shameful secrets.

Then and now

Advertising from the mid to late 20th century doubled down on these messages. From roller-skaters in pristine white clothes, to "mystery blue liquid" showing product absorbency, to packaging with no mention of "tampon" or "menstruation," themes of secrecy, hygiene, protection, and embarrassment were rife. It took until the mid 1980s for someone (Courtney Cox of *Friends* fame) to even *say* the word "period" in a TV commercial, and sadly—with only a couple of recent exceptions positioned as "activism" from the corporate manufacturers themselves—these themes are all identifiable in 21st-century advertising media.

How were our parents and grandparents taught about periods?

Today's older generations grew up a world in which much of life had already been marinated in consumer culture, including the education they received on the subject of menstruation.

For millennia, menstruators passed on what they knew about periods to their children, older siblings taught younger ones, and menstrual knowledge and management methods were handed down based on home and community resources and values.

Things changed in the 1920s and 1930s. To advertise the new menstrual products they were peddling (see page 20), companies reached out to mothers and daughters in free leaflets filled with scientific-sounding jargon, encouraging them to step into a bright new future of modern products. This information began replacing the intergenerational family conversations of the past.

As a generation came to rely on the new products, they trusted the accompanying corporate messages more and more. Over time, corporations realized that, if they reached out to schools, they could advertise to thousands of potential customers.

Captive audiences

In 1946, the Kotex brand partnered with Disney to create an animated educational film and a booklet that, together, became a full class lesson. These gave facts on menstrual anatomy and busted some entrenched myths, reassuring people that it was fine to exercise and shower during your period, for instance. Though factual and well-intentioned, this partnership led to other menstrual product companies following suit, offering in-house educational materials alongside free samples in an attempt to gain loyal customers from their first period. By ensuring their products and branding were emblazoned across the educational materials, corporate influence was embedded within educational institutions. Kids left those classes with brand recognition and an association of trusted knowledge with corporations, an introduction to all the insidious messaging woven into menstrual product advertising, and a focus on consumerism being the key to all things period. When they grew up and became teachers and parents themselves, and companies reached out to them or their kids, this practice seemed normal, and still continues in some form today.

Be wary of branding

If you find commercial branding on any health-based informative literature, check the data against alternative sources.

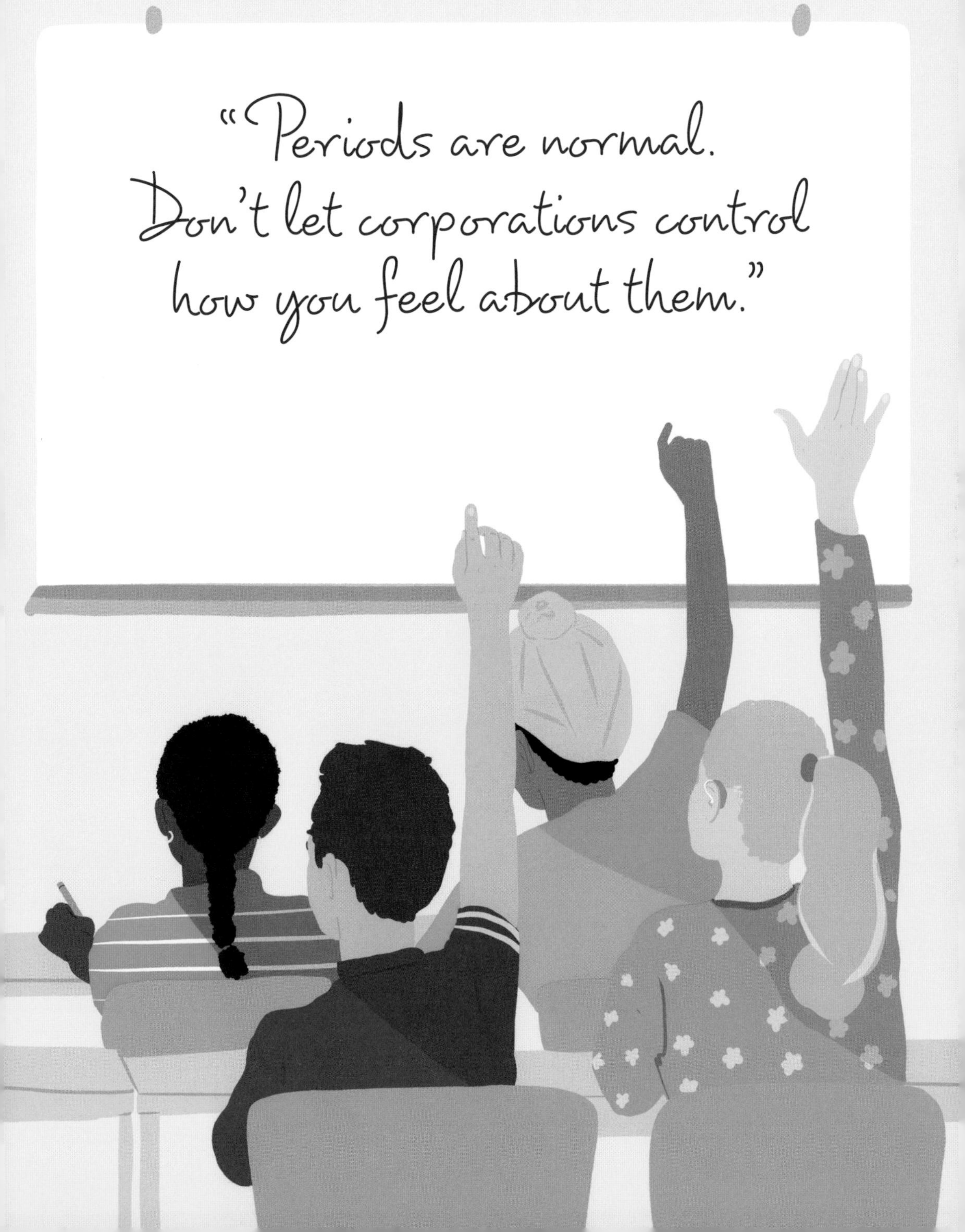
"Periods are normal.
Don't let corporations control
how you feel about them."

What are some longstanding myths about periods?

When you list the superstitions and myths about menstruation, past and present, it's easy to identify fear and confusion. Let's do some myth-busting to help prevent repeating our collective history.

So many myths, so little time. Where can I even begin? Let's start in the kitchen. Below is a list of unfounded warnings about preparing food while menstruating:

◊ **Don't make** tomato sauce—either the pasta kind or the ketchup kind.

◊ **Don't milk** a cow or whip cream, because you will make that milk or cream curdle.

◊ **If you** make mayonnaise, it will spoil.

◊ **Your bread** dough won't rise.

◊ **If you're** trying to make pickles, just give up.

◊ **Forget about** making sushi; apparently, your sense of smell is taking the week off.

◊ **Don't cook** food for yourself, and definitely don't cook for anyone else or you will poison them. In fact, don't even go into the kitchen!

And there are so many things that are bad for you (see opposite). But do you know what's good for you? Ignoring these old superstitions!

Why did these myths persist?

We can point a finger at the patriarchy here. Such beliefs, especially those suggesting that menstruation makes you poisonous, could often overtly, or covertly, control the actions and movements of menstruators. In the days before the scientific insight we have today, even experts played fast and loose with hypotheses concerning menstruation. But that's only part of the story. There was also a belief by healers in both the East and the West that menstrual blood being stuck in the body was bad for you. And don't forget the "wandering womb" theory (page 16)! Because of these concerns, based on the science of the day, any activity that might stop the flow or shake up the uterus was considered dangerously unhealthy.

Because of the taboo, not talking about myths meant that no one corrected them.

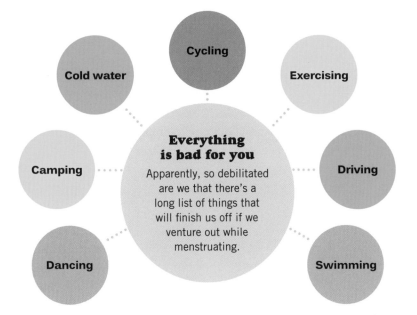

Cycling

Cold water

Exercising

Camping

Everything is bad for you

Apparently, so debilitated are we that there's a long list of things that will finish us off if we venture out while menstruating.

Driving

Dancing

Swimming

Even euphemisms for menstruation like "moon time" or "time of the month" that give the whole thing a lovely poetic feeling reinforce a few myths about periods that many people still believe today: that periods should happen once a month (although cycles can be longer or shorter), that we synchronize with the moon (we don't—it's purely coincidental if it seems like it's happening), and that the moon somehow controls periods (that's just the ocean tides, not the crimson tide).

Oh, and another synchronization myth that needs to be busted is the idea that the cycles of menstruators in close contact will synchronize with each other. As fun and reassuring an idea as it is, it has been disproved. Before long-running studies with participants in shared houses were completed, some theories about reasons for syncing were pretty outlandish themselves. One was that there was an "alpha" menstruator influencing everyone else, like so many menstrual marionettes being controlled by one period puppeteer!

In fact, *all* of the above myths have been disproved. And while we may laugh at some, we should remember that these menstrual myths still do us a disservice—the echoes of them linger in people's reluctance to exercise, go places, and do things on their periods. One thing we can do to combat myths is correct them. Another is to break the rules constantly in some sort of permanent rebellious experiment.

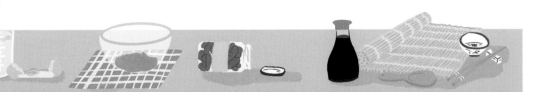

Why are periods still taboo?

Good question! They shouldn't be. Attitudes have changed so much in relation to, say, sexual health and gender equality, that it's frustrating the conversation hasn't moved on at the same pace when it comes to menstruation.

We now know so much about anatomy, biology, reproduction, the human genome.... We may not have flying cars yet, but we do have smartphones and commercial space flight. We are living in the future. So why are some attitudes to periods still so out of date?

Living in the past

It's down to a combination of everything we've discussed so far. The momentum of commercial menstrual product advertising and its influence on our language and purchasing habits (see pages 20–21), combined with education on menstruation being tied into those advertising tactics (see page 22), has interfered with the trajectory of our menstrual wokeness in a huge way. But now we have a chance to undo that damage and redirect this trajectory.

Periods are still taboo, essentially, because our global society is reluctant to let go of familiar old ideas, even when they don't serve us. We are still afraid, for the most part, to explore our own bodies fully and to talk about our medical worries and our fears of getting older. We don't acknowledge and address how taboos and myths (see pages 16 and 24–25)

Reclamation

Shame-laden influences imbued the idea of periods with negativity. It's time for menstruators to reclaim the conversation about this natural process.

often ended up subtly—or unsubtly—exerting influence over our fertility.

The fact that commercial menstrual products are unsustainable also triggers our fears, feeding into society's avoidance of looking at the environmental damage we cause. We have accidentally become entrenched in unsustainable systems in a counterintuitive doubling down that hurts us even more. But change doesn't have to hurt. We can treat ourselves positively and kindly as we learn and grow together.

Perpetuating the invisible

It's hard to notice menstrual taboos, because they are hiding in plain sight, and if you don't actively think about them and address them, you inadvertently perpetuate them. When menstrual myths and taboos are perpetuated, they become a hidden curriculum that we pass down to each new generation through school, in conversation, in movies and television shows, and in jokes and memes. And when taboos based on misunderstandings of menstruation are ubiquitous, they can cause individual and collective internalized shame.

Unnecessary euphemisms

Euphemisms for the word "menstruation" may have been used to minimize discomfort in conversations or save face, but they keep menstrual stigmas alive by maintaining the idea that periods shouldn't be talked about openly. So many euphemisms used around the world have a negative ring to them, subtly reinforcing the idea—even in jest—that we shouldn't talk about periods because they are dirty or evil or some kind of violent invasion. *The devil, the curse, the red army, code red, the red plague, a crime scene, bad luck, the Thing, Bloody Mary, the vampire, the monster, the crimson tide, the flood, the sacrificial ox*... Kind of explicit, no? And there are many more. There are also more benign phrases, like *Auntie Flo, my friend, the painters*

EUPHEMISMS
REINFORCE THE MESSAGE THAT YOU SHOULD AVOID USING THE WORD **"MENSTRUATION"**

are in, and *time of the month*. These may seem harmless, but their use reinforces the idea that we should be secretive about periods, which, by the way, is a euphemism itself—it's short for "menstrual period." These euphemisms also imply that the word "menstruation" is only for specialists, when really it's for everyone. And so the subject remains taboo. What can we do to reclaim our red stuff and menstruate with pride? Read the next chapter!

Break out of the negative cycle

Society's menstrual taboos lead to internalized shame about periods in individuals, creating negative personal attitudes to menstruation, which then feed back into societal attitudes. It's hard to recognize this feedback loop, break out of it, and release ourselves from the shame—but reframing it with period positivity disrupts the cycle.

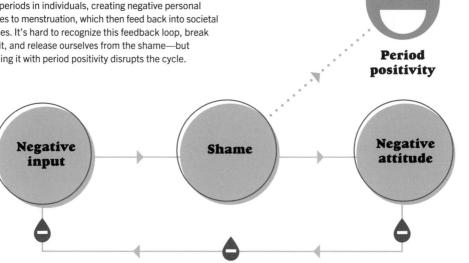

Period positivity

Negative input

Shame

Negative attitude

Period positivity

Once we discover how to recognize the media messages that tried to steer us wrong, being positive about periods becomes a piece of (red velvet) cake! You'll know how to talk about periods, ask questions when you're worried, reclaim leaks, bust myths when you hear them, and ensure every type of menstruator is included in the discussion. That way, menstruation becomes the normal, natural part of everyday life that it should be.

What is period positivity?

Period positivity is the practice of actively challenging the cultural discourse on menstruation so that it's no longer one of silence, shame, or embarrassment.

Transforming attitudes is never easy, and the best place to start is with ourselves. Ask yourself questions that help you identify negative ideas you hold about periods (see pages 20–27). For instance, how did you first learn about periods? Did the adults around you seem knowledgeable or nervous? Has talking about periods ever been awkward? Have you ever hidden your menstrual products or changed your behavior because you were worried about leaking? Once you've recalled sources of the negative ideas you've absorbed, it's time to reframe them—we can do that together.

Get to know your period

Are you worried that your period isn't "normal"? Are you putting up with heavy flow because you think you have to? Are you afraid of blood stains? You're not alone—echoes of past attitudes influence how we feel today. One way to undo this is to chart your cycle (see pages 90–91). Recognize it for what it is—a normal bodily function and a vital sign that you're healthy and that your body is working well.

Don't be afraid to talk

Do you avoid conversations about periods with nonmenstruators or use euphemisms or gestures to refer to all things menstrual? Consider period talk a bit of solo activism! Once you start to discuss your cycle with friends, partners, or colleagues the way you'd talk about movies or current events, you can draw parallels between experiences and compare notes. It's exhilarating once you start! Soon enough, you'll be asking older generations about their experiences and serving as an example to younger people in your life. When we share, we challenge outdated ideas together.

Tackle internalized shame

This is a tough one, but it's the most important. Do periods make you feel uneasy? Have you absorbed messages that periods are dirty? Internalized shame (see page 33) is an awful feeling. It can hold you back from making confident decisions and feeling happy and healthy. The shame twists your thinking to make you feel as though periods are something bad that your body does or something awful that "happens" to you—as though you are "naturally shameful." And you are absolutely not!

Exercise choice

When it comes to menstrual management, did you ever buy the most expensive menstrual product because it was at eye level on the shelf, or maybe it was recommended by educational pamphlets given at your school "period talk"? Have you supported a brand because its ad linked it to a charity or activism? Do you think of a particular product as being old-fashioned, for someone richer or poorer than you, or just for "someone else"?

Do you worry people will judge you for the products you use? You don't have to follow the crowd, accept advertisers' messages, or use just any product offered to you. There are more options than you'd think (see page 62). You have the agency to make an informed choice about what works for you.

Contribute to menstrual literacy

You don't have to become a campaigner to make a difference. Being period positive is about changing your attitude and using that leverage to elevate the attitudes of others around you. How will you change your self-care to support your own healthy menstruation? What changes can you initiate at work or school? How can you reclaim the menstrual narrative from corporations? Every positive step nudges this global conversation in the right direction, and as you explore your knowledge and feelings about periods, you're making a bigger contribution than you think!

Might I have been taught misconceptions about menstruation?

Buckle up, because yes. Heck yes. Remember when I told you our parents and grandparents had their menstruation education hijacked (see page 22)? Well, those problems are still with us.

Some misconceptions have been passed on by parents sharing what was taught to them, with little idea they were misguiding you.

In schools

Teachers often relied on biased resources that were sponsored by menstrual product manufacturers. And until very recently, lessons in some religious schools avoided teaching about tampons—a ridiculous vestige of the notion that tampons somehow interfere with virginity.

Often in schools, the period talk remains just that—one talk rather than a lifelong discussion or a series of "teachable moments" outside of class time. This discourages us from seeing periods as a topic for everyday conversation.

In the media

Most reported scientific research in the news media, and even a lot of activism, is conducted or funded by the companies that make menstrual products. Robust data is hard to come by unless you know where to look—like university outreach, public engagement initiatives, or by reading health journals.

Covert messages

Some misconceptions are passed on stealthily, picked up as incidental knowledge from ads, packaging, and society at large. For example, you may have absorbed the received "wisdom" that periods should be hidden, that your cycle should be exactly 28 days long, or that boys shouldn't know about periods. You may have internalized the idea that nonmenstruators are better than menstruators. And you've almost certainly picked up the idea that leaking menstrual blood is a social disaster.

MENSTRUAL CONCEALMENT

Researchers point out that some menstrual discourses and policies that seem positive at first actually focus on what they call "menstrual concealment."

This is the idea that menstruators should hide, manage, or stop menstrual blood to always appear as a nonmenstruating person. What we need instead is to shine a light on corporate overinvolvement in public attitudes to periods. We need discourses that help increase menstrual literacy, focusing on cultural knowledge, science, and body awareness. We need acceptance of the fact that there will be blood, that it may sometimes be visible, and that our choices about concealing it—or not—shouldn't be commodified.

How can we get rid of menstrual shame?

Internalized shame isn't easy to spot. You may feel you have a positive attitude to menstruation, but if you are holding onto shame deep down, it can govern your feelings and behavior.

If you harbor negativity about menstruation, it affects both the big and the casual choices you make, the subjects you talk about, how you see and care for your body, and aspects of your relationships. To replace this shame with pride takes self-inquiry, so brace yourself. If visceral feelings of fear, discomfort, embarrassment, or anger arise, shame may be hanging around, too.

Assess your menstrual education

How did you learn about menstruation? Was your primary educator knowledgeable and confident? If they seemed hesitant, you may have internalized their embarrassment, making you feel inhibited. You might believe myths, ignore your gut feelings, and defer to others, who may dismiss your worries.

If you were never taught about periods and were terrified when yours began, you may have decided that periods are scary, dangerous, to be kept a secret, and wrong or bad—and that you must be wrong or bad for having them. Such feelings make people even more susceptible to the negative messaging in ads (see pages 20–21) and, often, less likely to seek medical help.

Trust yourself

Beyond self-inquiry, the first step to rid yourself of internalized shame is to remember that your body is powerful, that it does interesting stuff, and that anyone who implies that periods are something to be embarrassed about is wrong.

Once you've identified your deep menstrual fears, try to look at them objectively. How do you feel about them when you're not worrying about how you *think* you should feel? The best way to challenge shame is with joy. The joy of learning, the joy of humor and art, and the joyful camaraderie of sharing with friends will all be helpful to you on this journey. You have it in you to become your own best advocate.

Why is it important to say "menstrual products" and not "feminine hygiene"?

Well, because "menstrual" is what they are. There's nothing unhygenic about this awesome thing our bodies can do, so the word "hygiene" is misleading. And who's to say how "feminine" you are?

The phrases "feminine hygiene" and "sanitary protection" didn't turn up in our collective vocab until the disposable menstrual product industry started using them to help sell their products (see pages 20–21). We know the sanpro industry has played fast and loose with our feelings over the decades, using taboos and fears to urge people to buy their stuff. These terms frame menstruation and menstruators as dirty, and by using them, advertisers were able to keep generations of consumers buying their products for the "protection" they afforded from the apparently disgusting horror that was periods.

But the thing is, other products that are used for cleaning up after bodily functions aren't framed in the same negative way. For instance, diapers are advertised as diapers, not clean-bottom diapers, and tissues are simply tissues, not boogerless-nostril tissues. So why does this one product get singled out to push the fear-and-self-loathing factor in advertising? Why do we need to be constantly told that people think periods—and only periods—are dirty, and that we might leak "unhygenic" menstrual blood at any moment without their "safe," "leakproof," and "discreet" products?

"Feminine"?

Whatever your gender or gender expression, companies shouldn't use outdated language or ideals to frame who you are as a customer.

Don't buy it

When it comes to these phrases and the products that they describe, I decided years ago that, both figuratively and literally, I just don't buy it—and I invite you to join me in this dual linguistic and consumer boycott. I don't accept that just because "sanitary" or "feminine hygiene" have been around for a hundred years, they are my tradition. They don't add up to a valuable piece of lore that's been handed down the generations. Their use is nothing more than outdated, manipulative advertising lingo, which has no place in my vocabulary, body, or bank statement. Instead, I buy brands that have moved on from this language, and I say "menstrual products". After all, the words "menstrual" and "menstruation" are not just for doctors or scientists—they're for everyone. So say "menstruation" with pride!

"The words we use are powerful—
they influence our thoughts.
Choosing and using them
carefully is period positive."

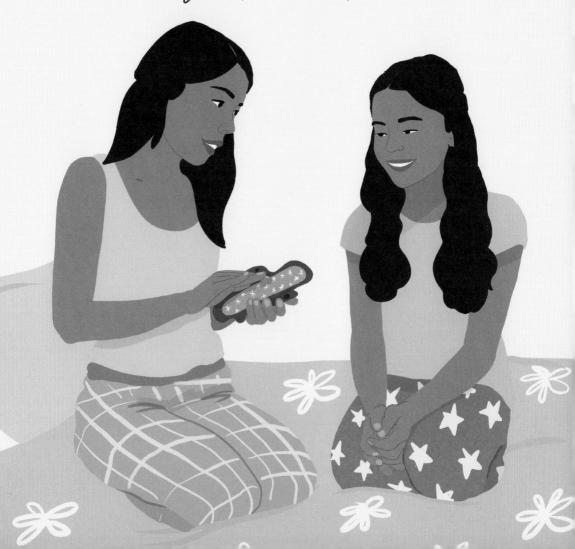

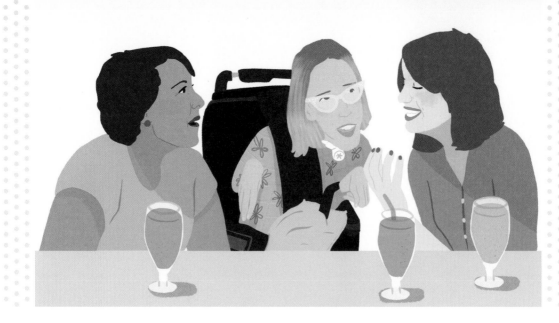

Does period positivity mean all periods are great? Mine aren't!

Let's be honest—periods can be a real pain in the uterus. Period positivity is being informed enough and confident enough to advocate for what you need.

Period positivity is not about all periods being awesome. What *is* awesome is the group enlightenment that takes place when we talk openly about periods. As we emerge from an era in which people have kept menstruation a secret, even from other menstruators, taking steps to remove this stigma is period positive.

Period positive action

Even if your periods are problematic, actively managing the issue is a period positive action. Period positivity means talking to your friends to compare notes about periods, and if you find

yours are atypical, talking to your doctor. It means charting your cycle (see pages 90–91) to gather useful data to share with them to help resolve your problem.

When people use the phrase "period positivity" incorrectly, it can make others believe that it frivolously implies that you shouldn't complain about your period or that the period positivity movement exists in name only and requires no effort. In reality, it takes effort to break through barriers of years of embarrassment and shame and being taught social norms that go against what's right for our bodies and minds.

Why is it important to say "menstruators" when I talk about people who menstruate?

Everyone who menstruates has a stake in the menstrual discourse. If menstrual policy, research, and media affect you, they should include you.

Many people presume that anyone who presents as a woman menstruates and that anyone presenting as a man doesn't. However, this isn't necessarily the case. A lot of trans and nonbinary people who don't choose to medically transition will still get periods and regularly navigate managing them in ways that align with their gender and gender expression. Trans-inclusive reproductive health conversations often incorporate reclaimed or reimagined vocabulary to support this.

It's also important to remember that not all women menstruate due to anatomical, medical, or hormonal reasons. Also, some menstruators are intersex, some people haven't started their periods yet, and some have stopped having them. So it's more inclusive to avoid only using the phrase "women and girls" when what you really mean is people who have periods.

Whether you get periods or not shouldn't define you as a person. It's an aspect of life that links to complex feelings—around gender, around fertility, around shame, around aging ... elements of our identities that are being rediscovered, reexplored, and reclaimed before our eyes—with incredibly empowering results.

Never underestimate the way language can act as a gatekeeper for who's in and who's out. When we're talking period positivity, everyone who menstruates is most certainly *in*.

Gender-neutral terminology

Using the term "menstruator" or the phrase "people who menstruate" makes it very clear that menstruators come in all forms. It also encourages us to ensure all menstruators are included in groups, conversations, advocacy, and education that directly impacts all of us. If someone hassles you about it, assert that you're advocating for everyone who gets periods, not just the majority.

Cycling together

It's more accurate and inclusive to use gender-neutral terminology to truly represent the full spectrum of people along for the ride.

I belong to a marginalized group. Does this impact me as a menstruator?

If you're a menstruator from a group that's marginalized in society, you may face specific barriers. It's important to identify these issues and take practical steps to address them.

Systemic inequalities have an impact on many issues, and this answer is by no means exhaustive. And menstruators on the margins can even be overlooked by campaigns and policy initiatives.

You may find that a doctor, colleague, or even a friend makes assumptions about your experience based on bias or stereotypes, unconsciously or consciously. Microaggressions can derail your whole experience of periods. Bucking taboos to talk about menstruation takes effort, and it can be energy sapping to deal with intersectional oppressions (experiencing more than one type of discrimination based on identity or circumstances).

Be alert to any suspected discrimination around seeking contraception, termination, or fertility treatment. Below are situations to look out for, questions to ask, and practical suggestions for navigating difficult circumstances.

Neurodiverse menstruators

If you are sensitive to rough surfaces or clothing tags, consider the materials you find comfortable when choosing menstrual products. You may wish to opt for reusables over disposables.

Periods can be difficult to manage if you are overwhelmed by overstimulation or a change in your routines. Try to build in downtime and develop strategies for times when PMS impacts your usual coping mechanisms. If you experience executive function issues, look at period tracker apps that remind you to log data or smart thermometers for cycle charting (see page 91). Use your phone calendar to set alerts for changing/washing/carrying products.

Survivors of assault and trauma

If you have PTSD or have experienced trauma, especially if it relates to your sexual or reproductive well-being, managing menstruation or reproductive health can be triggering. If you have flashbacks or panic attacks during routine procedures, or fear you might, confirm in advance that medical staff will use protocols for treating trauma survivors and request a support attendant.

Menstruators and mental health

Ads for menstrual products have a lot to answer for (see pages 20–21). Negative language can reinforce body shame and fear, and encouraging secrecy can make it difficult for people struggling with body image, anxiety, or an eating disorder to manage their periods without feeling triggered. Understanding the messaging is key to helping you break free of its influence.

Be aware that OCD symptoms can flare up during periods or be exacerbated by PMDD (see page 99). PMDD can be misdiagnosed as bipolar disorder or depression. Track your cycle, linking your symptoms to it, and use this evidence to press specialists to investigate further if you think there's more to it.

Menstruators with reduced dexterity

Some conditions or physical disabilities such as dyspraxia, cerebral palsy, or EDS (Ehlers-Danlos syndrome) affect mobility or fine motor control, making it difficult to insert and/or remove internal menstrual products.

Recently, there have been innovations in menstrual cup design by disabled inventors to improve the way cups can be used one-handed or with limited dexterity. Look for a cup made of ultra-pliable silicone with a loop-style pull tab for easy grasping. You can also get tampons with a looped string.

Remind doctors and nurses to communicate directly with you if they habitually address your partner, carer, or assistant.

Menstruators of color

Despite increased awareness of institutional racism, it still lurks in our health systems. For example, "pain bias" (when reported pain is not taken seriously by a healthcare provider) is something experienced by women of color in particular, who find their reporting of pain is minimized or dismissed. This can lead to symptoms of endometriosis being missed and has been logged as a potential contributor to preventable maternal deaths.

If you feel your doctor is dismissing your concerns, question it or find another doctor.

LGBTQIA+ menstruators

Although menstrual and reproductive health management is becoming more queer-inclusive, there's a long way to go, particularly for trans inclusion. Ask for menstrual products and step trash cans to be provided in gender-neutral and men's toilets at your place of work. Use inclusive language. Challenge bi erasure in family-planning settings. Share your pronouns at clinic visits. Seek out menstrual products that feature designs or advertising targeting a variety of gender expressions.

Menstruators of size

Menstrual products can and should be designed to suit the needs of people at every size. Seek out brands selling pads and period underwear in larger sizes and ask other companies when they'll be stocking them. Don't be afraid to advocate for yourself with healthcare providers: people can be fit at any size, and doctors should not base decisions solely on BMI or assume all fat menstruators are unhealthy.

Tone policing

Don't be surprised if your assertive complaint is mislabeled "aggressive." Join forces and seek advocacy from groups specific to your needs. Self-advocacy fatigue is real.

What is a period positive school?

It is a school where everyone, from students to the principal and superintendent, through all the teaching and counseling staff, to the lunch and janitorial staff, are trained in menstrual literacy.

In a period positive school, there will be a staff and student team responsible for ensuring that the environment, facilities, curriculum, and activities all have menstruators in mind and for making changes where required. These schools aim to improve the way we talk about menstruation in society as a whole by positively influencing the conversation within and beyond school grounds, improving the discourse for staff; parents; and, most importantly, students.

The future of menstruation education

All staff should be trained and ready to explain something period-related in a teachable moment or give out a menstrual product as the need arises. A period positive school teaches kids all about fertility and menopause, too, to provide full knowledge on menstruating bodies. And of course, the school will develop their own resources with trained and trusted staff and not allow their menstruation education to be dictated by the companies that sell menstrual products, or use imagery or resources linked to brands.

It shouldn't stop there, which is why I set up an award along with my research. Schools must develop ongoing conversations about menstruation as part of human resources and include it in teaching wherever possible. For instance, home economics students can make their own reusable pads; math students can explore the stats of menstruation; and English or communications studies can teach the use of persuasive language in ad campaigns for menstrual products. Imagine if *our* schools had been like this.

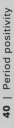
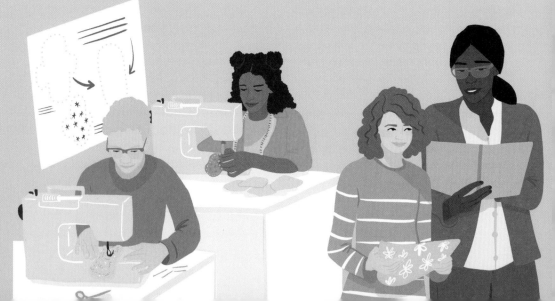

What is a period positive workplace?

A period positive workplace is one that has fair policies and practices for all staff, with an environment that is inclusive and also supports staff who menstruate throughout their menovulatory lifetime.

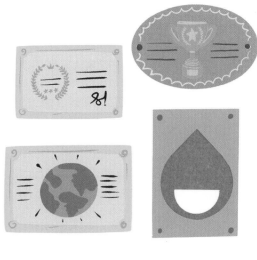

Employers hoping to create a period positive workplace should first try to create a fair and ethical workplace for everyone, with fair pay and hours, safe conditions, supportive absence policies, and clear paths to promotion or leadership roles. Next, they should ensure that managing periods doesn't feel like an added stress or something to hide. Knowing you can talk about reproductive health at work, whether privately with your manager or casually with colleagues, can take a load off your mind. When it comes to period-related matters, many employees actively self-edit these topics, worried about how the conversation will be received, or because of internalized menstrual shame (see page 33).

A company that writes a menstrual-leave clause into its HR policy indicates to employees that period talk is welcome talk. Policies should incorporate all aspects of reproductive health and provide assurances that issues at any stage of our reproductive lifetimes can be accommodated. You may hear arguments like "separating out menstrual leave can increase the stigma, so people should just use sick leave," but it's more nuanced than that. Periods aren't

a sickness, and if symptoms regularly require several days' leave, you should investigate the underlying cause. However, hormones do make our energy levels cyclical, and flexible working policies can support this. How do we get to that point if people are suffering in silence? The first benefit to a policy is visibility.

Turning the tide

Many companies are introducing menstruation and menopause policies. Don't be afraid to request necessary or helpful policy changes. Audit your workplace environment—for instance, in the bathrooms, is there a cubicle with a sink and a trash can so you can wash a menstrual cup or throw away used disposable products conveniently? Are there adequate bathroom or rest breaks? Is there an exception to a repeat-absence policy when those absences coincide with an employee's menstrual cycle? Don't be afraid to ask your employer to look at this stuff. People used to worry that it made menstruators seem weak or would hold them back, but that attitude doesn't stand up today, as more employees are advocating for their rights—menstrual and otherwise.

How should we talk to nonmenstruators about periods?

Frequently; openly; confidently; and, if at all possible, with humor. Nonmenstruators are as curious as we are about periods but have often been left out of the conversation altogether.

You may need to overcome your own embarrassment as you wade into a conversation about periods with a nonmenstruator, but you should quickly find it's worth the effort, as they are often grateful for the candid chat.

Don't presume that the nonmenstruators you meet aren't as woke as heck. Many of them recognize how much a part of life it is for a menstruator and are curious about the experience, but they have not had access to reliable information. They may have presumed or even been told all kinds of odd stuff and would appreciate being set straight.

And you also shouldn't presume that everyone you think is a nonmenstruator actually is, or you might accidentally menses-splain periods to a seasoned bleeder! But there are plenty of nonmenstruators out there who you may end up talking to who want—or need—to know more. This might be a partner, a colleague, a younger sibling, your dad, your 4-year-old nephew ....

Just dive in

If they ask you a question and it's a person and setting that feels comfortable and safe for you, answer it. If it's a case of "right person, wrong moment," try and have a quick reply for the short term so you can talk more when you feel less "on the spot." If you don't answer it, and it's someone you know well or who looks up to you, you might accidentally transmit to them an association between periods and secrecy or shame.

A lot of us have a tendency to self-edit around people who don't menstruate. Let me tell you that nonmenstruators don't need protecting, and we deserve to be surrounded by people of all genders who know all about the menstrual cycle. After all, none of us would be alive without it. More folks than you realize have a healthy respect for the menstrual cycle and are eager to find out more.

Start with their experience

A good starting point for discussion is asking questions. How did they first learn about periods? How knowledgeable do they feel now? Their answers will be telling.

How can we teach younger generations to be period positive?

It's important not to shy away from the subject of menstruation when kids ask. Most of their questions can be answered with age-appropriate information.

A good place to start thinking about how to teach children to be positive about periods is to think about what we wish we'd known before we started puberty … and then go back even earlier. Kids can be taught about

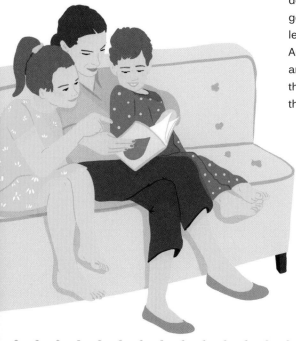

periods as soon as they're old enough to see menstrual products in the bathroom, or have a parent who is pregnant with a younger sibling. Three-year-olds already know about pee, poop, boogers, and vomit. They can handle learning about periods. So if a young child asks you about menstrual products, explain in a simple way what they are. If they ask about what that red stuff is, tell them it's the blood that bodies can make to protect a baby in a person's tummy like a big cozy blanket—or something like that. They're just curious.

Normalizing puberty

As kids get older, we should teach them about periods early on in elementary school. As soon as they can learn about cats having kittens or the water cycle, they can conceptualize what periods are. For the few children who start puberty early, it will be such a huge relief for them to know that periods are not something they should feel awkward about and that it doesn't have to be a great big secret. Kids of all genders should be taught together so everyone learns about the variety of puberty experiences. And it should happen far enough in advance, and with enough candor, that it isn't framed in their minds as a horrible, suspenseful thing that is looming ahead.

And, of course, for this positive message to really embed in the minds of children, it can't be a one-time thing. Menstruation needs to be talked about at home, at school, in the community, and beyond, so that kids grow up to pass the message on, too.

Blood

Menstrual blood is often presented as scary, dirty, and embarrassing, but what actually is it? Overcome any blood fears, or stock up on facts to help others deal with theirs by reading all about it—what it's made of, where it comes from, how much there should be, and ways to manage it. You'll also find out what you should expect from your cycle, plus what to do if you discover that *your* normal is actually pretty unusual after all.

Is menstrual blood the same as other blood?

Blood is blood, but by the time it leaves your body, menstrual blood also includes endometrial tissue and other components.

Menstrual blood comes from the endometrial layer. It is the blood inside the many blood vessels that form part of the endometrium, which provides a welcoming surface for a fertilized egg to implant itself into and a nutrient-rich layer for a placenta to hook onto. As the endometrium sheds the top layer of its lining each cycle, the blood vessels break down, and the blood and tissue are released from the uterus. As blood leaves the body, it collects other stuff that affects its color and consistency.

Menstrual blood contains vaginal secretions, cervical mucus, and endometrial tissue, and it tends to be darker in color than venous blood. You may also see clots. Menstrual blood also contains fibroblasts (cells that produce proteins that help make blood thicken) and platelets (little parts of blood cells that help form clots). These all add up to produce menstrual flow with colors and textures that may make it seem a little different in appearance to, say, a nosebleed.

Consistency and flow

The consistency of menstrual blood can change across your menstrual cycle and throughout your menovulatory life (see page 114). Blood may be anywhere from light pink to bright red, thicker darker red, or brown (see page 54), and you may have small or larger clots in it (see page 55). It will look different on different surfaces (on your underwear, on your fingers, in a menstrual cup, on a pad, and on toilet paper).

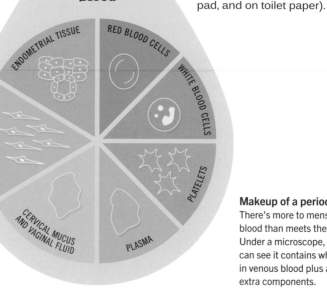

Menstrual blood

ENDOMETRIAL TISSUE

RED BLOOD CELLS

WHITE BLOOD CELLS

FIBROBLASTS

PLATELETS

CERVICAL MUCUS AND VAGINAL FLUID

PLASMA

Makeup of a period
There's more to menstrual blood than meets the eye. Under a microscope, you can see it contains what's in venous blood plus a few extra components.

How do I get over a fear of blood?

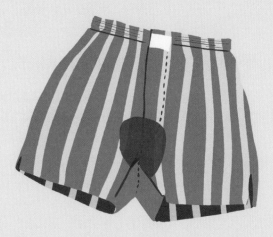

First of all, give yourself a break for having this fear. There's so much negativity around periods and menstruating bodies, it's hardly any wonder people can be scared of menstrual blood. You are not alone.

If people don't feel comfortable with the idea of menstruation or feel uncomfortable about touching their own bodies, how their vulva looks (see page 48), or how their reproductive organs work, they are less likely to feel comfortable with menstrual blood, and vice versa. It's about the taboo itself for many people rather than the actual bodily fluid. Someone with a fear of menstrual blood might feel fine dealing with a bloody nose or watching a horror movie.

Pin it down

Try to identify the causes of your fear. For instance, when you were young and fell and scraped your knee, you may have learned to connect bleeding with being hurt. Or maybe you're worried about germs or by the idea that menstrual blood is a potential germ carrier? Are you grossed out by all bodily functions? Do you feel uncomfortable putting your fingers in your vulva or vagina? And do you have leakage fear? Did you have an awkward

school or work period stain incident that you haven't forgotten? Understanding the nature of your fear can help you develop strategies to move beyond it.

You'll get there

First, try taking a look at a menstrual product you've just used. Next, explore your vulva and vagina while you're having your period (maybe a light day at first, then a heavier flow day next cycle). If you avoid certain menstrual products because you worry about touching your blood, try switching it up. Blood is a bodily fluid, so you should follow the usual sensibilities of washing your hands before you leave the bathroom, but otherwise just keep reminding yourself that it's your own body, after all. You can teach yourself that you are nothing to be afraid of.

> ### Feeling faint
>
> For some people, fainting at the sight of blood (vasovagal syncope) is a quirk of the body's autonomic nervous system, and it's just one of those things—not shame-related at all.

What does a "normal" vulva look like?

The question should be "What *doesn't* a normal vulva look like?" I'm serious. The fact is, if you've seen one vulva, you've seen *one* vulva.

Below is an example of a vulva, labeled with all the parts, but—and this is crucial—this is not the only vulva on earth. No vulva you see in a book is going to be exactly like yours, and your vulva will change as you age. What's more, your vulva is not your vagina. Feel free to correct people when they get this wrong. It may contain the vaginal opening, but the vulva is front and center, and when you naming it to reclaim it feels good.

So now that we know the vulva is a unique body part, let's look at this unavoidably generic "everyvulva" to see what's what. The hood and glans of the clitoris, the perineum, and the labia (outer and inner) are sort of your north, south, east, and west. In the middle, from top to bottom, you've got the urethral opening and the vaginal opening, with some more sensitive structures just under the surface.

Labia

You may have seen labia labeled *majora* and *minora* (Latin for "bigger" and "smaller"), but

"Everyvulva"
While vulvas come in many shapes, sizes, and colors, vulval anatomy is roughly consistent.

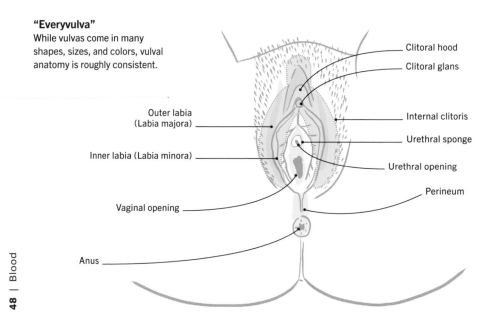

Clitoral hood

Clitoral glans

Outer labia
(Labia majora)

Internal clitoris

Urethral sponge

Inner labia (Labia minora)

Urethral opening

Vaginal opening

Perineum

Anus

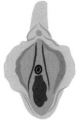 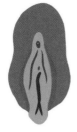 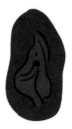

Labia
Labia—also known as "vaginal lips"—come in all shapes, sizes, and colors.

many sources now use "inner" and "outer", refering to the "bracket" shapes labia make from your thighs inward. But this can be confusing, because for some people, the inner ones stick out farther forward than the outer ones, while others' inner labia can't be seen because their outer labia are ... let's say, pursing their lips. Labia may or may not be symmetrical. And you definitely don't need to "improve" the natural color, size, or shape of your labia. Don't let anyone convince you otherwise.

The clitoris
Now let's move up to the clitoris. Did you know that the clitoris is gigantic? It may be cute as a button on the surface, but beneath the skin, there is a lot going on that medical science didn't know about until alarmingly recently! The internal length and breadth of the clitoris means that, if you want to have an orgasm, there are many places you can stimulate that will still be rubbing the clitoris up the right way. Giving you orgasms is the only thing that this friend-for-life organ is for. How good is that? Add in the urethral sponge and perineal sponge—tissue under the skin that engorges at arousal—and you can see why different types of vulval stimulation can be so pleasurable.

Pubic hairstyles
Vulvas can be hairy, and that hair is valuable. It helps protect the microbiome of your vagina from external particles. For some people, vulva hair covers only a little bit of space above or around the labia, and for others, it covers a lot of the pelvic area. It's also totally normal for it to extend onto your thighs and/or up your belly.

Don't feel you have to trim, wax, shave, or otherwise style it unless you want to, but if you do, be kind to your skin, which can become easily irritated or infected in this sensitive area.

A word on discharge
Healthy discharge takes several forms, but may all look the same in your underwear: a bit of white, clear, or creamy staining when ovulating or aroused. This is normal and a sign that your body is working well! The vaginal microbiome is naturally acidic, so it may bleach the gusset of your underwear—also totally normal!

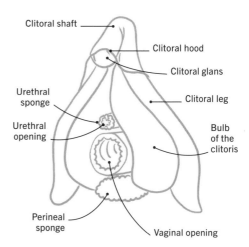

Clitoral shaft

Clitoral hood

Clitoral glans

Urethral sponge

Urethral opening

Clitoral leg

Bulb of the clitoris

Perineal sponge

Vaginal opening

The structure of the clitoris
The clitoris nearly encircles all of the parts of the vulva and can be stimulated from many directions as a result.

"When it comes to periods, 'normal' usually means what's healthy and typical for you."

How much blood is a normal amount to lose?

The amount of blood lost during a period does vary from person to person, but, in general, it's probably less than you're imagining, and it usually leaves the body slowly.

The average amount of blood to lose during the course of a period is 2–6 tablespoons. You should be able to find a product that has the absorbency to keep you going for a few hours at a time before you need to change it, and you probably won't experience leaks very often. If you're not sure how much blood you lose, use a menstrual cup (see pages 66–67) to help you keep a running tally across one period, or count the number of times you change other types of product. If you suspect that your periods are too light or too heavy, see pages 52–53.

"Flobbalobba"

This is the word I use to joke about that big rush of period blood that happens now and again if you've been in one position for a while.

Expectations

Many menstruators only have a vague idea of what a period is actually like before it first happens. Often, this was not explained well at the school "period talk." Kids don't generally realize that bleeding during your period is a gradual affair. In reality, it's usually more of a trickle than a flood, yet many kids nervously expect a scene from a horror movie!

Because menstrual cycles are irregular at first, by the time they settle down, someone struggling to manage excessively heavy bleeding may become desensitized, believing that this level of flow is typical, particularly if they were predisposed to expect a lot of blood. The lack of information and open discussion of periods doesn't help. People can end up suffering in silence for years, with no idea that there could be a medical explanation for their excessive bleeding.

We often talk about "heavy days" and "light days," and it's common to experience a great big *flobbalobba* of blood escaping in one go when you sneeze or get out of bed in the morning. But you shouldn't be bleeding lots and lots of blood over the course of each cycle—if you are worried, or if you notice a significant change to your flow, seek medical advice.

Is it okay if my period is really heavy or really light?

Everybody's flow is unique to them, but if yours seems to have settled at either of the extreme ends of the spectrum, it's worth discussing with a doctor.

Your flow will settle into a pattern, if it hasn't already, and will probably remain consistent for years (see page 142). The amount of blood you lose in a period can vary throughout your life as hormone levels shift (usually postpregnancy or as you're approaching menopause), but, in general, you will have your own personal normal, and it may be lighter or heavier than others'. If there is a sudden change in either direction, though, see your doctor.

Where it becomes less subjective is when the quantity of blood you lose during each period is outside of the normal range. Estimate how much blood you're producing (see page 51 for tips), then compare your findings to the information in the table below.

Seek reassurance

For a long time, people were discouraged from talking about periods (see pages 20–21), and many felt very alone with their worries. Lately, though, as we break the taboos surrounding menstruation, more people are opening up and comparing notes. Such reassurance is invaluable—seek it out if in doubt!

Of course, some people have a better idea than others of what to say when they want to talk to friends, relatives, or even complete

What is "too light"?	What is "too heavy"?
A flow that is "too light" is one that results in less than 2 tablespoons, or 30 ml, of menstrual blood across the course of one cycle. In this case, it may be that your body is not producing enough hormones for the uterine lining to grow (see page 87). It could also be a sign of pregnancy. It is worth seeing a doctor to get to the bottom of the issue.	A flow of more than roughly 6 tablespoons, or 80 ml, across one period is considered "too heavy." You might find you're changing menstrual products much more frequently than others are or often bleeding onto clothes or bedsheets. You should definitely see a doctor if this is the case, as it is possible you have a period-related hormone imbalance or a medical issue such as endometriosis (see page 106) or fibroids.

strangers about periods. If you want to bring it up, you could start with something along the lines of "I'm on day two of my period and it's always really heavy—are you the same?" If you're at the other end of the flow spectrum, you could try "My friends get jealous when they find out I have really light periods and can sometimes go without any products at all toward the end—anyone else?" Both are great opening gambits that friends tried with me before I became "Period Girl," and both led to supportive discussions.

Conversations like these help change people's attitudes toward period talk. Being more open allows us to notice when we have stuff in common with our friends. This can also lead to earlier diagnoses of medical

YOU HAVE A **HEAVY FLOW** IF YOU NEED TO CHANGE MENSTRUAL PRODUCTS EVERY

1–2 HOURS

problems, as fewer people will suffer in silence or feel too shy to stand up to any doctor who doesn't listen.

Ultimately, mutual understanding will force advertisers to stop using shame or scare tactics to sell their products, as they will no longer work.

Measuring flow
Flow is often measured in tablespoons. Using a menstrual cup is the easiest way to visually "measure" your period.

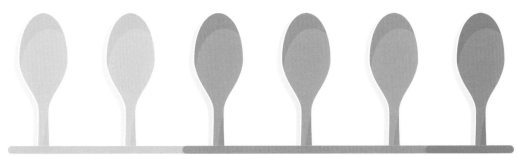

Light flow

Average flow

Heavy flow

Less than 2 tablespoons across the course of one cycle is too light

More than 6 tablespoons across the course of one cycle is too heavy

Why does blood change color over the course of a period?

Menstrual blood comes in a range of shades. There's usually a simple explanation behind each change in color.

How old or how thick menstrual blood is influences its color, as do other bodily fluids that mix with it. These are fairly typical reasons for color variation and are usually nothing to worry about.

Light in color

Let's start with the lighter end of the spectrum. Menstrual blood can be pink at the start or end of your cycle if you are spotting due to lower estrogen levels (say, if you're perimenopausal or on the pill) or if it has mixed with cervical mucus, which is white or clear.

Bright red

This blood is the freshest and usually flows at the beginning of your period. Some people only have bright red period blood but, like all blood, it will become darker once it leaves the body.

Bright red blood between periods may not be normal. It can be a sign of injury, infection, or cancer, so please get that investigated right away if it occurs.

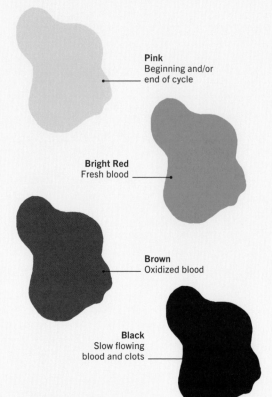

Pink
Beginning and/or end of cycle

Bright Red
Fresh blood

Brown
Oxidized blood

Black
Slow flowing blood and clots

Light to dark
Comparing the color of your blood across your period, you'll probably notice it varies widely.

Darker blood

Now let's move over to the dark side. Blood becomes darker as it comes into contact with the air and oxidizes, so what flows out as bright red may have turned into a brown stain by the time you see it on a pad, in your pants, or on your bedsheets or clothing. If your blood is flowing very slowly, it may start to turn brown as it leaves the body.

Clots (see opposite) can also be very dark red in color, sometimes appearing almost black.

Should I be worried if I see clots?

Although blobs in your blood can look a little scary at first, be reassured that many people get them and they aren't usually cause for concern.

Clots appear as dark globs of blood. They are, essentially, very thick blood that has sort of jellified. All blood in the body has the capacity to coagulate (thicken), which helps reduce blood loss if you have a cut. In the case of blood from the endometrial lining, this useful attribute performs another function—it helps build up the lining of the uterus during each menstrual cycle (see page 87). I like to think of it as your body creating a nice comfy duvet inside your uterus to prepare for a future guest.

Clots can look kind of gross or kind of interesting, depending on how you feel about blood. If you're not squeamish, next time you have clots in your menstrual blood, try squishing one between two pieces of toilet paper. You'll see that it leaves brighter red stains on the paper. Clots are made up of many layers of bright red blood, but the layers are so thick that they appear dense and almost black. Squishing one enables you to see how thick they are. Aren't bodies great?

When to be concerned

It's worth getting clots checked out if:
- **They appear** suddenly and you've never had them during your period before.
- **You are** struggling to deal with very heavy flow and you have many clots simultaneously.
- **The clots** seem very large (bigger than a 10¢ coin).

Thicker texture
Larger clots may be visible on pads or in a menstrual cup, but there's usually no need to be alarmed if you see them regularly.

How can I manage leaks?

The best way is by refusing to feel shame. After all, despite societal aversion to seeing menstrual blood, it's a normal part of life.

Let's deal with the practicalities first. It can certainly be uncomfortable if your period starts and you don't have any menstrual products on hand or if you feel yourself overflowing on a particularly heavy day. To avoid discomfort, bear in mind the following:

◊ **Track your** cycle (see pages 90–91) so you know roughly when you're due to have it.

◊ **If your** cycle is irregular, look for signs that your period's due, such as cramps, or count 14 days from when you noticed signs of ovulation (see page 89).

◊ **Carry your** preferred menstrual product(s) during the day or two on either side of your expected period in case you start early or bleed longer than usual.

◊ **Use the** right product, size, or absorbency for your flow, varying it as needed.

◊ **Consider other** variables, like whether you'll be traveling or stuck in one location for a while without being able to change your product.

Reframe your thinking

Remember that no product is 100 percent leakproof. Fish gotta swim, birds gotta fly, periods gotta period—and that's just fine. The idea that leaking is a terrible disaster is so last century—don't buy into it! Imagine how different each day of your period would be if you just didn't care. Consider all the adjustments, big and small, that you make in order to avoid leakage and all the energy spent worrying about leaking.

When you think about it, it's not periods that interrupt your day so much as all the worrying about keeping them concealed. The period positive way to manage periods is with the bored nonchalance evident in our management of every other normal bodily function. After all, hiding your periods is bad for your self-esteem. So if you do leak, try making a deliberate—defiant—choice to not die of embarrassment while you handle the practicalities. However you choose to deal with the situation you find yourself in, I invite you to do it with style. You'll often find that others follow your lead.

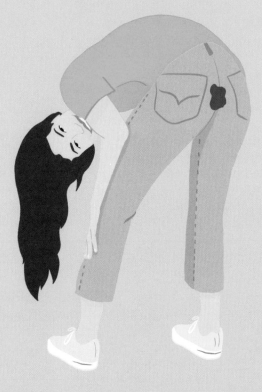

What's the best way to deal with period stains?

For your well-being? With confidence, nerve, and a healthy dose of humor. For your clothing and soft furnishings? With speed, precision, and cold water.

As a menstruator, blood stains are par for the course, just as ketchup stains are for those who love ketchup and lipstick stains are for lipstick wearers! If you treat them as the normal occurrences they actually are, you encourage other menstruators to do the same. That said, it also pays to be in the know on easy cleaning methods.

Removing stains

As soon as you can, remove the item of clothing that you've bled on and soak it in cold water. (Avoid hot water!) I'm not saying you should do this in the office kitchen sink, but the sooner you get the garment soaking, the better. Give it a gentle scrub or rub it with some stain remover if you can, then stick the item in the wash the same day with whatever else can go into that load, on a cold wash cycle. Heat is not your friend here. Then hang the fabric to dry—using a dryer may set any stain that remains.

Embracing stains

As I said, heat is not your friend, including the heat that may be rising in your cheeks when you realize you've leaked, if you harbor embarrassment about public leaking. It's time to retrain your brain about the stain.

Do you remember my slumber party story (see page 6)? That experience eventually made me actively change the way I reacted to leaks and stains—and I'm not alone in this. Many menstruators are fed up with feeling humiliated by outdated perceptions about our bodies simply behaving like our bodies. So if you find you've permanently stained a favorite garment, turn it into a cloth pad design and—take it from me—don't lose any sleep over it.

What are the pros and cons of disposable menstrual products?

When single-use menstrual products were first invented, they were a game changer, but this innovation is now literally costing us the earth.

Despite recent inroads into more eco-friendly choices, many people are still of the mindset that disposable menstrual products are a necessity and that the plastic-based ones in particular protect us from leaks.

So stuck in this mindset are we that disposables are often the first thing we reach for. So it's worth stopping to consider their pros and cons and weighing, with more consideration, what factors you'd like to include in your choice of menstrual products.

The pros

There is one major pro with disposables—their convenience. In some situations, it's not easy to make use of reusable products. For instance, if there is no sink in the bathroom cubicles at work or school, a menstrual cup is messier to empty, rinse, and reinsert. But there is usually a trash can provided for tampons and disposable pads.

Also, it's not always convenient to carry around used cloth pads or period underwear in a wet bag throughout your day or evening so you can take them home to clean them. Sometimes periods come early and you need a solution while out and about. And depending on where you live, work, or visit, the plumbing and clean water infrastructure may not be robust enough to meet your needs for washing reusables safely.

So disposables might be your best bet if you need a no-effort option. All you have to do is buy them and throw them out. But this convenience comes at a cost. Several types of costs, actually.

The cons

If you *do* have options, think about how many disposable products you might go through in a single period, then multiply that to account for 35–40 years of menstruating. A store's own brand may be pretty cheap, but if you're buying the premium brand products that are relentlessly marketed to us, the price adds up.

They are also unsustainable. Disposable products harm the earth through the harvesting of the raw materials required to make them, the use of ecologically unsound ingredients such as plastic top sheets and gel inserts, and the plethora of plastic packaging—sometimes layer upon layer of it.

There's no denying they come with a hefty carbon footprint. Energy is required to produce

4.3 BILLION
DISPOSABLE MENSTRUAL PRODUCTS ARE **USED PER YEAR** IN THE UK ALONE

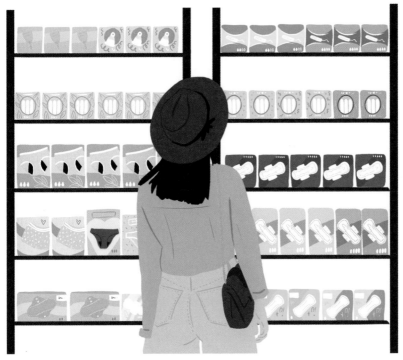

Purchasing power
Even if you access free products, you still have a choice over which ones. If you want to use reusables, make this clear to the product provider.

the raw materials and then manufacture and package the products in factories, and that's all before the big multinational companies that make them ship them around the globe.

And on top of all of that, they create a huge pile of garbage—about 11,000 disposable menstrual products per person end up in landfills, while countless tampon applicators and wipes wash up on beaches and clog sewers.

Seek out more ethical options

If you need the convenience of disposable menstrual products, you can choose more ethical options. You can ensure your disposables are chlorine-free and plastic-free and made of organic unbleached cotton or bamboo.

Consider the packaging, too. Is there an unnecessary amount of it? Is it made using sustainably forested wood and plant-based dyes? Look out for tampons with no applicator or an applicator that's made of cardboard or PET plastic or is reusable. Seek out pads wrapped in paper, or those that come loose in the box rather than individually wrapped in plastic. (You can carry them in a small container when you're out and about.) And check the place of manufacture of a product to consider its air miles.

There are many smaller companies leading the way with responsible menstrual product practices. Hopefully, bigger corporations will one day follow suit! See pages 60–61 for solutions that involve reusables.

Why are people moving toward sustainable menstrual products?

Consumer culture is changing as more and more people choose to buy sustainable products, whether for environmental or cost reasons.

Until the 1920s, reusable menstrual products and natural materials were the be-all and end-all of menstrual management. Isn't that wild? Over the last century, clever marketing convinced just a few generations of us that we couldn't cope without disposable menstrual products (see page 20–21). Well, that's a load of nonsense!

Sea change

In the atomic age of the mid-20th century, people had visions of the future that we now

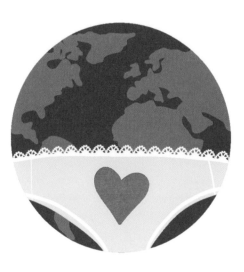

think of as a bit over the top and kitschy, especially when compared to how things have actually turned out. Back then, to be "modern," things had to be quick, shiny, and super-convenient. Throwaway culture was the height of fashion. But what's becoming clear to us in the 21st century is that speed and convenience did not give people more leisure time but instead have made people consume more, and therefore have to work more to pay for more. And that has come with an environmental cost, too (see pages 58–59).

Now, thankfully, we are beginning to unlearn throwaway culture. We've begun giving up paper plates, polystyrene packaging, and plastic cutlery; swapped single-use coffee cups for reusable travel mugs; and started to ditch plastic shopping bags. Some places have welcomed a tax on disposable products and have started looking critically at fast fashion in our favorite stores.

Amazingly, it took a whole lot longer for us to start talking about the problems with disposable menstrual products. Just as many "essential" products have been superseded by more sustainable choices, the tide is turning on menstrual products too. We're heading back to the land of reusables, but now with added innovation.

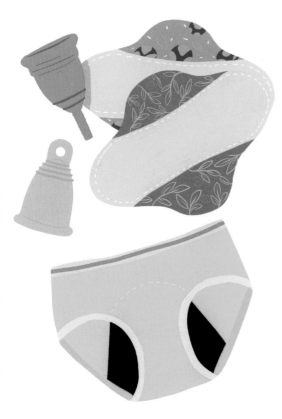

better value, especially if you're on a low or no income. But they are definitely cheaper in the long run and worth saving up for, if possible.

Many brands offer refunds if you don't take to their product. There are also programs in some areas that subsidize the cost of reusable menstrual products or distribute free ones. When choosing, consider how ethical the manufacturer's practices are, including what sizes they cover, their advertising messages, and whether they spend their profits pushing their product to kids in schools (see page 22).

CONSUMER POWER
IS VALUABLE AND
SHOULD NOT BE UNDERESTIMATED

Purchasing ethical products

The market for reusable menstrual products has been growing swiftly since 2015. More and more people, institutions, and organizations are starting to teach about them, promote them, and consider them. Period underwear (see page 64), menstrual cups (see pages 66–67), and cloth pads (see page 65) in clever designs and new technologies are taking us back to our period-history roots in a really good way.

Purchasing reusable products does involve more of an initial outlay than tampons or pads. When you see reusable products on the shelf in the same store as disposables, it might be hard to convince yourself that the upfront cost is

Keep an eye out for small companies that make or distribute ethically sourced menstrual products of all types—you can support a local business at the same time. Alternatively, you could make your own cloth pads. If you have the resources, it's really not that difficult (see page 65), and you'll get even more satisfaction out of using sustainable products you've made yourself.

How do I choose the right menstrual product for me?

We all have unique needs, and our choice of menstrual products will reflect that. So when choosing for yourself, don't settle—put *your* preferences first.

You can choose from the whole range of menstrual products. This can depend on your practical needs, a preference for one type you love using, or a focus on sustainable products, if that is your main priority.

Mix and match

Some people become accustomed to using the same product all the time, but you may choose to use a mix, depending on where you are and what your plans are for that day.

For instance, you might use cloth pads at home because they're comfortable and easy to soak and wash when convenient. Or you might find period underwear best for a day's work or study, as you don't have to change them often.

For a day at the pool or a night on the town, an internal product might be more practical. You might even choose to pair an internal and external product for a heavy-flow day.

If you're traveling, you might be happy to use whatever products are available locally, or you may feel more comfortable bringing enough of your own preferred products for the duration of your trip. When camping, you could use a menstrual cup, sterilizing it in a pan on a camping stove, or pack a few pads or tampons (and take any trash with you when you leave).

Each type of product comes in different shapes and sizes, and many have a range of absorbencies, too.

Whatever you choose, know that there are many products out there. If you feel your menstrual needs haven't been met yet, you may not have found the products that work best for you. Keep trying different styles to find what you need, or invent your own!

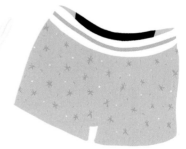

"You deserve an informed choice about what products will serve you physically, financially, and ethically."

How do period underwear work?

Like a dream! When you find the size and style that works for you, you'll want to wear a pair every day, even when you don't have your period.

In the simplest terms, period underwear is underwear with a pad inside the fabric. The reinforced gusset section is made up of a breathable, moisture-wicking top layer that sits against your body, absorbent inner layers that catch most of the blood, and a moisture-resistant bottom panel to stop the blood from escaping.

Many people find period underwear preferable to pads. The blood never leaves the gusset area, they rarely leak or even drip, and they feel comfy, not bulky, to wear. Period underwear usually feels and looks just like normal underwear in most aspects of the design other than the gusset and center sections. Different brands offer various colors and styles, including boy shorts and sporty looks.

Build the right set

As well as the standard "daytime" pants, there are period underwear for nights and others for light days. Nighttime types have an additional circle of reinforcement extending backward from the gusset up to the waistband—making them perfect not just for sleeping in, but also if you're a back bleeder or your flow is heavy. Pants for light days have fewer or thinner internal absorbent layers.

The initial outlay may be high, but you'll have savings in the long run. You could start by buying just one or two pairs, but remember that they take time to wash and dry. If you want to use pants throughout your period, you will probably need about five or six pairs—it's likely you'll get through two to three pairs per day.

Practical matters

Wash period underwear with your clothes as normal, then hang them to dry—clothes dryers warp their shape and diminish their absorbency.

They will eventually become less absorbent over time. Different brands provide varying estimates for the lifetime of their underwear. Even though the gusset may bleach or discolor over time, they should all last for a few years.

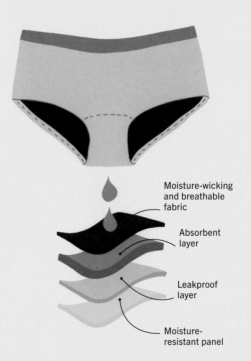

Moisture-wicking and breathable fabric

Absorbent layer

Leakproof layer

Moisture-resistant panel

How can I make my own reusable menstrual pads?

If you have access to the resources, making cloth pads can save money and reduce your contribution to landfills.

Sewing your own pads is easier than you might think. There's even a global network of pad makers sharing advice, patterns, and video tutorials online. You can always keep things simple in the spirit of our ancestors, who successfully used folded fabric remnants without any fancy construction for millennia (see page 18). Making pads is also a nice way to reuse a favorite old pair of pajamas, a towel, or a robe that's seen better days.

Fabrics and designs

The most basic pattern is a rectangle or circle that you simply fold up or sew in short stacks to create layers, then position around the gusset of your underwear so it is the thickness you need that day.

You'll need a few different fabrics with specific properties: something soft and moisture-wicking that's safe against skin, such as organic cotton; something hyper-absorbent like bamboo fleece; and a waterproof layer, such as combination cotton and PUL. Ensure you sew the layers together rather than using iron-on adhesive fabrics, which are non-absorbent. You can make your pads with wings and add a method of closure (such as snap fasteners) to keep them securely in place.

Get creative
Use cute shapes or fun printed fabric for your pads to really make them your own.

How do you use a menstrual cup?

Way more easily than you'd think—it won't take long to get the hang of it. And there are a bunch of good reasons to use one.

Not only is using a menstrual cup convenient, but it also minimizes your environmental impact and saves you money by eliminating or drastically reducing your use of disposable menstrual products. While a cup may cost a bit more than disposables initially, it will pay for itself within several months and last for years.

Because they're made of medical-grade silicone, menstrual cups feel more comfortable against the walls of the vagina than tampons. And, unlike tampons, silicone doesn't absorb your vagina's natural lubrication, so you experience less or no uncomfortable dryness.

What's more, because cups catch (rather than absorb) blood, using one enables you to easily monitor your blood loss across your period. This means you can quickly recognize heavy and light flow days and spot changes to your bleeding pattern that might indicate a medical problem. Some cups even have measurement marks on the sides. Don't use a cup if you have an IUD fitted—it may cause your IUD to get dislodged.

Choosing a cup

Finding the right cup may involve some trial and error. Pelvic floor muscles help hold the cup in place, so it's useful to know how strong yours are (see page 76) so you can choose a cup that's likely to fit you well. Larger sizes are better suited to people with weaker muscles, including those who have given birth vaginally.

Cups come in different shapes, too. Some may fit your unique anatomy better than others. Once you've tried a particular shape, if it's uncomfortable, you'll have a better idea of what to try instead.

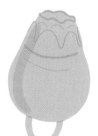

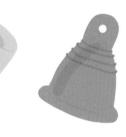

Finding your fit
Some cups are wider at the top, while others are the same width nearly all the way down. The rim may be wide or flat. Stems can be long or short and shaped like a stalk or ring.

Using your cup

Before using your cup, sterilize it according to the manufacturer's instructions. If you've never used one before, try it first on a heavy-flow day—your blood will act as a lubricant, helping you insert the cup. (Don't use actual lube, as it interferes with the cup's suction seal.) If you've used tampons before, you'll get the hang of this in no time.

Ensure your hands are clean before insertion. You'll need to fold the cup's rim so that it fits into the entrance of your vagina. There are a few nifty techniques you can use, two of which are shown here (see right).

Insert the folded end into your vagina and push the cup in. It needs to be placed high enough to allow you to sit comfortably and so none of it sticks out. (You may need to trim the stem.) It will unfold once it's in the right position, with its rim pressing gently against the vaginal walls. To help it form a seal, you may need to wiggle it from side to side, or pull it down slightly until you can feel that it's fully open and in place.

How often you need to empty your menstrual cup depends on your flow. With a light flow, you can leave it in place for up to eight hours safely; any longer increases the risk of overflowing and, in rare cases, TSS (see page 72). To remove it, insert a clean finger into your vagina and hook it over the cup's rim to break the seal. Now, using the stem, gently pull out the cup, keeping it level so the blood doesn't spill. Tip the blood out into the toilet or sink, rinse the cup if you can (using cold water first will prevent stains), then reinsert it in the same way. Be sure to sterilize it at the end of your cycle before storing, ready for the next month.

A menstrual cup should last for up to ten years, but if you see that the silicone is starting to degrade, replace it sooner.

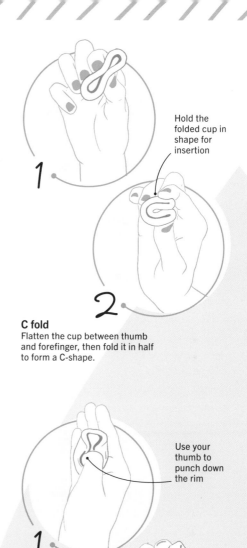

1

Hold the folded cup in shape for insertion

2

C fold
Flatten the cup between thumb and forefinger, then fold it in half to form a C-shape.

1

Use your thumb to punch down the rim

2

Punch down
Push one section of the rim into the cup, then pinch the sides together around the punched-down section.

I'm afraid of tampons. How do I use them?

Many people find the idea of inserting something into their vagina uncomfortable at best, terrifying at worst. If you want to give it a try, read on.

It's important to undo any hang-ups you might be harboring about tampons. Vaginal muscles can tense up involuntarily, and when the vagina is tense, it's difficult to push anything up there.

The best thing to do is relax as far as possible and just try inserting a tampon a few times. It also helps to understand the shape of the vagina (see opposite). See how it's angled backward, not upward? When putting in a tampon, push it in at that angle, rather than straight up. Follow the advice opposite for positioning it correctly.

APPLICATOR OR NOT?

Tampons come either with or without an applicator—which option is better?

If you're new to using tampons, some people recommend beginning with the applicator types. However, you'll find it easier to trace the contour of your vagina using your index finger and an applicator-free tampon. If that works for you, keep at it. If you find your finger is too short, then seek out a tampon with an applicator (preferably a plastic-free one). With either type, it's important to wash your hands before inserting.

Practice insertion

If you're trying to use a tampon for the first time when you have your period, your menstrual blood will be the lubricant that helps the tampon slide into your vagina without friction. If you'd rather try when you're not having your period, you will find it more comfortable to use actual lubricant to practice, rubbing a

IF TAMPONS DON'T WORK OUT, TRY A CUP. A LOT OF FOLKS FIND THEM EASIER BOTH CONCEPTUALLY AND PRACTICALLY.

little on the tip of the tampon and applicator. Bear in mind that lube decreases the absorbency of tampons, so it should not be used when you have your period. And note that tampons usually sit higher than cups in your vagina. (You should never use silicone-based lube on a silicone product, so don't try this with a menstrual cup.)

Go ahead and tear through a whole box of tampons if you need to, to help familiarize yourself with inserting them, feeling for the string, and removing them. You may waste a pack, but you'll gain a skill.

What is the ideal positioning for a tampon?

If your tampon isn't comfortable to wear, it's probably not in the right position. Once you get the hang of it, you'll be able to insert one by feel without even thinking about it.

Vaginas average between 2½ and 4 inches (6 and 10 cm) in length. The outer two-thirds are the most sensitive, particularly because the bulbs of the clitoris extend beneath the surface here. But the farther back you go, closer to the cervix, the less sensation there is. This makes the back third of your vagina a good place in which to position a tampon—you're less likely to feel it if you sit awkwardly, if you need to pee, or if your vaginal muscles involuntarily tense up.

Placing tampons high in the vagina is also practical. Menstrual blood exits the uterus via the cervix, so having the tampon close by, ready to absorb it immediately, makes sense.

Know your own anatomy

It helps to have a sense of the proportions you're working with, so insert a finger into your vagina and have a feel around. Then, once you have a sense of the length of your vagina, try inserting a nonapplicator tampon to get an idea of how much space it takes up. Stand up straight, walk around, sit down, and see if you can feel the tampon. If you can feel it, try gently pushing it in farther, or remove it and start again with a new one. Once you feel comfortable, you've most likely positioned it correctly.

And don't worry about a tampon getting "lost" up there. If you can't get one out, you might be tensing up, so try to relax as you pull the string.

Practice makes perfect
To get the tampon position right, get comfortable before inserting it—whether sitting, squatting, or standing.

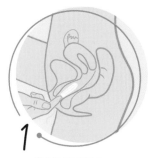

1. Put in a tampon, pushing it gently to the back of your vagina.

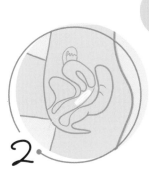

2. If it's in the right place, you'll be comfortable.

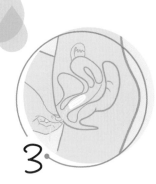

3. Pull on the string to remove the tampon.

What can I do when I don't have any menstrual products on hand?

For a start, don't panic. There are easy ways of improvising a temporary fix. But before we get into those, let's think about that panic for a second.

People have been having periods forever, so why does this feel like a crisis? Changing your attitude to leaks (see page 56) will banish the fear—you can choose to not care and bleed away!

That said, stains can be inconvenient and wet underwear uncomfortable, and there are situations in which free bleeding isn't possible. Try asking others around for a product—friends, colleagues, and strangers are often happy to help. From a talk at the sinks to a general call from a stall, don't be afraid to cast a wide net. If you have no luck and there are no vending machines in the bathroom, there are temporary fixes.

Handy substitutes

Make an improvised pad with a paper napkin surrounding a wad of toilet paper, tissue, or paper towels. A slightly less absorbent outer layer won't get soggy and fall apart as quickly. Don't use paper products to improvise a tampon: they might leave fibers behind in the vagina, which could cause an infection. And remember: these are short-term fixes that should only be used until you get a hold of your preferred products.

You can also add a layer of clothing over or under what you're already wearing to bleed into. Avoid staying overdressed for too long, though. Air needs to circulate well near your vulva to protect the microbiome of your vagina.

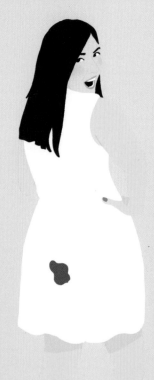

Go with the flow
If you get "surprised," you can simply do nothing—by choice rather than as a last resort. Free bleeding, if done by choice (see page 18), can be empowering.

What if one pad or tampon isn't enough?

You're not alone if you have a heavy flow (see pages 52–53). If you regularly find that one product at a time is not working well enough for you, there are options.

First, consider switching products. It may be that you will benefit from the full coverage of heavy absorbency period underwear or nighttime pad designs. Also, some brands are better at handling heavier flow than others, so try out different styles to see if you can find one that meets your needs.

Doubling up

Have you tried doubling up? Try a combination of internal and external products—use either a tampon or menstrual cup internally, then a pad or period underwear externally to catch the overflow.

You can also use two pads if you don't get along with internal products. This is a useful (if slightly wasteful) hack for overnight, if you don't have any extra-long nighttime pads. Position one pad toward the front of your underwear and one toward the back, with the ends overlapping over the gusset. If you need to change them frequently, you can leave the mostly unused ends exposed and just add a fresh pad over the middle. You should probably only do this once, though—more will likely be uncomfortable. Never use two tampons at the same time.

Check the absorbency

If you find you're consistently buying products with inadequate absorbency, check the packaging to determine how much blood the product can hold. Each package of disposable menstrual products displays an absorbency indicator. Look for a little row of pad or tampon outlines, with some of the shapes filled in and some left blank. More of the shapes will be filled in for products with greater absorbency. Don't use tampons with more absorbency than you need, though—doing so puts you at increased risk of toxic shock syndrome (see page 72).

CONSIDERING A MENSTRUAL CUP?

A menstrual cup (see pages 66–67) can work wonders with a very heavy flow.

If you can get by with a cup and it's convenient for you to empty it frequently, it might be right for you, and will also save money longterm. Plus, if you're concerned about the environmental impact of using disposable products, it's reassuring to know that a cup is less wasteful.

What is toxic shock syndrome?

You may have been warned about toxic shock syndrome (TSS) at school. Cases caused by tampon use are rare but serious, so it's important to be aware of the risks and symptoms.

TSS is a medical emergency that is caused by bacteria entering the body and releasing toxins, leading to sepsis, which can be fatal.

Staphylococcus and streptococcus bacteria live on skin and in mucous membranes harmlessly. But if they are introduced into the body (through a cut, for instance) and increase in number, this can cause TSS. The situation can quickly become deadly. Toxins produced by the bacteria cause the immune system to go into overdrive, which can result in multiorgan failure. One way in which these bacteria can enter the body is by being transferred into the vagina on a tampon. The risk increases if any of the fibers from the tampon remain behind in the vagina when it's removed.

Symptoms of TSS

The symptoms can appear similar to those of other illnesses, such as a cold or flu. Symptoms include a high fever, headache, chills, exhaustion, a rash, bloodshot eyes, diarrhea, dizziness or disorientation, breathing difficulties, and fainting. It's extremely serious. If diagnosed early, TSS can be treated with IV antibiotics in hospital. If untreated or caught too late, it can lead to organ failure and death.

Although TSS is more associated with tampons, there have been very rare reported cases of a suspected link between TSS and menstrual cup use. As cups are made of medical-grade silicone, they do not shed fibers, so they don't seem to carry the same level of risk. You should not share your menstrual cup with anyone else, even if you sterilize it between uses.

REDUCING YOUR RISK

Observing the following measures will help reduce your risk of TSS:

- Wash your hands before inserting a tampon.
- Only use tampons at the correct absorbency for your flow—don't go heavier to try to buy more time.
- Change tampons frequently (every four hours whenever possible), and never leave a tampon in for more than six hours.
- Consider using other products at night.
- Only use one tampon at a time.
- Remember to remove the last tampon you use at the end of your cycle.
- Don't share menstrual cups with others.

How can I recognize vaginal infections?

Normal discharge is healthy (see page 49). But unusual discharge is one of several symptoms that often indicate an infection.

There are two types of infection. Some, such as bacterial vaginosis (BV) and yeast infection, are caused by the balance of the vagina's natural flora being out of whack. Others are transmitted sexually: for instance, chlamydia, herpes, HPV (see page 109), gonorrhea, and trichomoniasis.

If you notice any of the below symptoms, book an appointment with your doctor to investigate. It's important to seek treatment early—there's no need to suffer or feel embarrassed. There is an unnecessary stigma surrounding vaginal infections and STIs, but they are so common that there should be no judgment from healthcare practitioners when treating them. Depending on the type, vaginal infections are treated with oral and/or topical medication, and your doctor may advise a change to your self-care routine. If you experience repeat infections, ask for a referral to a specialist to investigate further.

There are several measures you can take to avoid vaginal infections. Wear breathable, loose-fitting underwear made of natural fibers and avoid wearing tights or synthetic leggings for too long. Stay hydrated and eat healthily—eating too much sugar or carbs can lead to yeast overproduction, causing yeast infection. Do not wash your inner vulva or your vagina, and avoid "feminine" washes, wipes, and sprays. Always have a pee after penis-in-vagina sex or using sex toys, and wash sex toys before use and share safely. See page 128 for advice on avoiding STIs.

Common symptoms			
Chlamydia	◆ Unusual discharge ◆ Lower abdominal pain	◆ Pain during sex ◆ Pain during urination	◆ Bleeding between periods ◆ Bleeding after sex
Bacterial vaginosis (BV)	◆ Unusual discharge ◆ Pain during urination	◆ Vulval or vaginal burning and/or itching	
Gonorrhea	◆ Unusual discharge ◆ Lower abdominal pain	◆ Pain during sex ◆ Pain during urination	◆ Bleeding between periods ◆ Bleeding after sex
Herpes	◆ Genital blisters or sores ◆ Pain during urination	◆ Vulval or vaginal tingling or burning	
Yeast infection	◆ Unusual discharge ◆ Pain during urination	◆ Vulval or vaginal burning and/or itching	
Trichomoniasis	◆ Unusual discharge ◆ Pain during sex	◆ Vulval or vaginal burning and/or itching	◆ Pain during urination
Syphilis	◆ Genital blisters, sores or painless ulcer	◆ Swollen lymph nodes	◆ Tiredness, aches, fever, and/or rash

My anatomy is atypical. Can I still use internal menstrual products?

It depends on the type of product and on your particular physiology. Ask your physician or specialist for advice, as everyone's internal anatomy is unique.

There are several reasons why some people are unable to use internal products. Bear in mind that, depending on your anatomy, it may be easier for you to insert a product than remove it.

Congenital conditions

There may be a physical barrier within the vagina caused by a congenital condition, such as a vaginal septum—a thin wall of tissue that divides the vagina into two. This septum can make it impossible to use internal menstrual products. In many instances, this can be addressed surgically if desired.

Weak internal musculature

Some medical conditions, such as certain types of Ehlers-Danlos syndrome, multiple sclerosis, or muscular dystrophy, can impact the tone of the pelvic floor and vaginal muscles, making it difficult to hold in a tampon or menstrual cup.

Support from a physiotherapist can help: they may recommend using exercises or weighted dilators to strengthen the pelvic floor. There are also menstrual cups designed for people with weaker muscles or limited mobility.

Scar tissue

Scar tissue resulting from surgery can change the size and shape of the vulva and vaginal opening. This can make using internal products uncomfortable. It's also recommended that you avoid internal products after some medical procedures, such as colposcopies (see page 109) and after giving birth.

FGM (female genital mutilation)

FGM can result in the near closure of the vulval opening and can leave scar tissue in the entrance to the vagina. This can block menstrual blood from leaving the body (hematocolpos), which can lead to infection. Some people who have experienced FGM also report more urinary tract infections and trauma around anything to do with their genitals. If you have had corrective surgery for FGM, avoid using internal products until the area has completely healed.

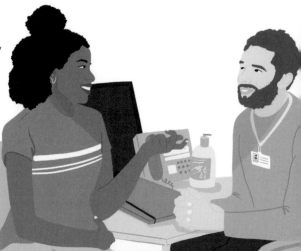

Am I the only one who finds internal products difficult to use?

No, you're not. Lots of people find them hard to use for practical reasons, as well as emotional and psychological ones.

For some folks, the shape of their pelvic anatomy makes using internal products difficult (see opposite). Others have mobility issues. For some, there are psychological reasons behind the aversion. Many people feel discomfort, shame, or fear when touching, talking about, or even thinking about their vagina. If this rings a bell for you, it's worth exploring these feelings, as they can stop you from getting essential medical check-ups, as well as affect your confidence generally. You deserve to feel positive about your body.

Vaginismus and trauma

Vaginismus is the fear of vaginal penetration. It causes the walls of the vagina to tighten involuntarily, which can impede the use of internal menstrual products, as well as penetrative sex. Ask your physician for a referral to a specialist. Physiotherapy and/or sex therapy may help.

Some causes of vaginismus can be addressed by understanding the cultural taboos and shame that we have internalized. Shame about menstruation or how our bodies look can be the main player here. Advertising has a lot to answer for (see pages 20–21). Start looking at

In the majority

Around the world, many more people use external products than internal. Even if your friends rave about internal products, if you prefer using external ones, remember you're in the majority.

body-shaming media critically and remember that every vulva is as unique—and beautiful— as every face (see pages 48–49).

However, there may be something going on that runs deeper than negative societal attitudes. Content notice: be aware that this next section could be triggering to read, so you may prefer to read it another time. Reluctance to use internal products might be linked to past trauma. If you associate your vagina with fear, shame, or panic, this may be due to memories of painful intercourse, unwanted sexual contact, abuse, assault, birth trauma, medical trauma, or gender dysphoria. It's important to process these feelings and seek help. There are many specialist services to which your doctor can refer you.

Fine motor skills

Health conditions that affect mobility or fine motor control can make it difficult to use internal products. Anything from dyspraxia to cerebral palsy to limb differences can impact the dexterity and flexibility needed to insert and remove products (see also left and page 39).

What are pelvic floor muscles?

Your orgasm-loving, trampoline-enjoying, baby-pushing-out, pee-holding-in pelvic floor muscles are your best darn pals.

Pelvic floor muscles are the ones you clench when you want to stop the flow of pee. What have they got to do with menstruation? Well, they enable your vagina to hold internal menstrual products in place, so if you like to use internal products, ensuring your pelvic floor muscles are in good shape is a good idea. And there are more reasons to keep them strong.

For one, a toned pelvic floor stops you from becoming incontinent. And another good reason for keeping them in shape is that they make orgasms better. As with any muscle, better muscle tone means better control. Orgasms are reportedly much more explosive when the pelvic floor is strong.

Pelvic floor weakening

Pelvic floor muscles can weaken with age, or due to injury during childbirth or sports, an increase in weight, or surgery. If you struggle with holding in pee when you sneeze or laugh, need to go frequently, or often feel a sense of urgency to pee, ask your doctor to refer you to a specialist physiotherapist. They will assess the strength of your pelvic floor on a scale of 1 to 5 and suggest appropriate exercises. They may also recommend an app or appliance to help you perform the exercises accurately and track your progress.

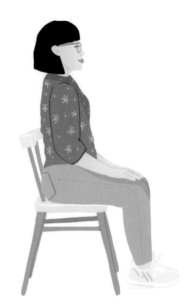

Pelvic floor exercises
You can work on your pelvic floor pretty much anywhere. One way is to sit upright and squeeze and relax your pelvic floor a few times.

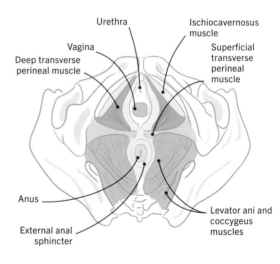

Urethra
Vagina
Deep transverse perineal muscle
Ischiocavernosus muscle
Superficial transverse perineal muscle
Anus
External anal sphincter
Levator ani and coccygeus muscles

Pelvic floor muscles
Your pelvic floor consists of several different muscles that collectively form a hammocklike structure surrounding your vagina, urethra, and anus.

Can I see the gynecologist when I have my period?

Sure! Most regular check-ups, IUD insertions, and Pap smears can be done at any time in your cycle, and doctors have seen it all before, so book that appointment and bleed away.

You don't need to worry about your doctor seeing your menstrual blood—these folks have seen every bodily fluid going! They've also seen lots of vaginas at every stage of a cycle. Besides—if you've been referred to a gynecologist for heavy menstrual bleeding, midcycle bleeds, or longer-than-average periods, your flow's not really giving you much of a "bleed-free" window there, and it's important to get it checked out.

Oh, and it may look like murder on the dance floor when you get up from the examination table, but chances are they stuck a big square pad down before you hopped on up there at the start of your visit, so no muss, no fuss—and no apologies needed. Maybe just mention you have your period at the start of the visit.

Cycle-specific visits

Some visits to the gynecologist for certain fertility or contraception-related matters need to happen at very specific points in your cycle, which might include during your period. If you're undergoing fertility treatment, sometimes you'll need a physical exam or to have blood drawn on a certain numbered day of your cycle. This is a common way to check things like your fertility, hormone levels, or whether you have ovulated during that cycle, or are about to. You'll be told if this is the case in plenty of time, and it's another good reason to chart your cycle (see pages 90–91).

Take charge of your health

Many people feel nervous at the idea of going to the gynecologist, but it's important to get the check-ups you need to stay healthy.

REMEMBER:
THE ONLY THING OLD TAMPON ADS GOT RIGHT IS THAT YOU CAN DO PRETTY MUCH ANYTHING **DURING YOUR PERIOD**

What do people in extreme situations do about their periods?

Whether you are climbing the world's tallest mountains, in the military, or orbiting the earth in a space station, periods still need to be considered.

Have you heard of Sally Ride, the first female US astronaut in space? When she was about to embark on a shuttle mission in 1983, a guy from Mission Control asked her if 100 tampons would be enough for the one-week trip! They didn't even check if her period was due. (It wasn't.)

Such cluelessness points to the fact that menstruators have historically been denied access to many jobs and opportunities. We have only recently become aware of what menstruators in extreme situations need and the potential pitfalls they face.

The fledgling research that exists tracks the experiences of menstruators across a number of fields, such as pro sports, the military, archaeological dig sites, and space travel. More research is needed on the physiological and emotional experiences and practical needs of menstruators in extreme situations.

Some research based on focus groups involving menstruators in the military has found that personnel often opt for hormonal contraception to suppress their periods (see page 100) for both practical menstruation management and contraceptive reasons.

Certainly, some people have unpredictable cycles due to the high-pressure environments and experiences they encounter. When you factor in long travel and few amenities, there is the potential for additional discomfort. For those using tampons with few opportunities to change them, there may be greater risk of toxic shock syndrome (see page 72). One thing's clear: there is an extreme need for more research.

Can I use diet and exercise to manage period symptoms?

What you eat and drink, and how much exercise you do, can have an impact on PMS and feelings throughout your cycle.

Having a diet that lacks essential nutrients, or not exercising much, might worsen some of the symptoms you notice around your period.

Try tracking your meals and activities alongside mood, menstrual symptoms, and the phases of your cycle for a few months (see pages 90–91). Your symptoms may correlate with changes to your exercise level, nutrition, sleep patterns, or calorie intake. Don't feel pressured to do this, though, especially if you have a difficult relationship with food. Be compassionate toward yourself.

Diet
Avoiding excess unhealthy fats and sugars and managing portion sizes is recommended for everyone, but it can be a particularly good idea to avoid heavy foods just before and during your period. This can help ease the sluggishness of sugar lows and carb overloading and reduce the tendency toward constipation that can happen before your period. Instead, eat a varied, high-fiber diet that includes all the recommended vitamins and minerals.

If you get PMS, avoid excess salt, sugar, trans fats, complex carbs, alcohol, and caffeine—the stuff you're probably craving. You may want something greasy, salty, and starchy, but if your periods or PMS are really bothering you, try your best to find a healthier option.

Ginger, peppermint, and raspberry leaf teas are all known to soothe nausea and cramps and are great for drinking during your period.

Exercise
You probably know that daily light exercise, more vigorous cardio a couple of times a week, and core- or strength-training routines are great for your physical and mental health. They also help relieve tension held in the abdominal and pelvic area and boost endorphins, which help with pain relief and energy levels.

If you find that your symptoms persist despite eating well and exercising regularly, it's worth seeing your doctor for advice.

"Your uterus is an expert at self-care: it knows when to have a good clear-out!"

What causes cramps?

Your awesome uterus, that's what. Cramps are a sign that the muscles of your uterus are pushing out its lining at the start of each cycle.

The uterus is strong. Really strong. It can stretch to accommodate a growing fetus and push out a baby. So when hormones stimulate it to shed the lining that's built up during a menstrual cycle, off it goes. See it as your uterus doing an excellent job at decluttering regularly. My uterus is more organized than I am!

Your body needs to get rid of the build-up of lining—if the lining of the endometrium kept building up without being shed in the course of each cycle, you could be more at risk of uterine cancer. (It's worth mentioning that missing periods due to hormonal birth control is *not* the same thing—see pages 120–121.) Cramps are what makes the blood come out.

A regular thing

In the absence of a pregnancy, estrogen and progesterone levels fall (see pages 86–87), causing the uterine lining to start shedding. When the soft outer part of the endometrium is not needed to nurture a pregnancy, the body expels it by contracting the uterine muscle fibers. This is a reflex action meant to remove irritants, which can include, in some cases, a dislodged IUD! The top layer of lining and blood separates from the endometrial tissue, and the uterus contracts over and over again to push it out through the cervix and vagina.

Cramps usually become more manageable after the first two days of your period. Track this and see what happens for you. You should find that toward the end of your period, when most of the blood has been expelled, cramps will lessen, then stop altogether. It's normal to feel cramps in your vulva, lower abdomen, lower back, bowels, or inner thighs. And you may also feel a twinge in one ovary at ovulation (see page 112)—this is called mittelschmerz.

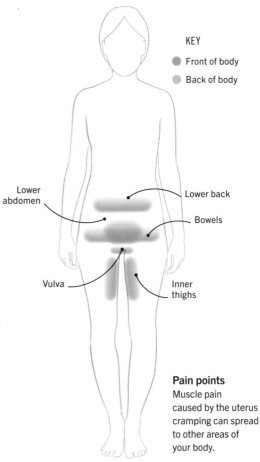

KEY

● Front of body
● Back of body

Lower abdomen

Lower back

Bowels

Vulva

Inner thighs

Pain points
Muscle pain caused by the uterus cramping can spread to other areas of your body.

Can orgasms help with menstrual cramps?

Yep! Think about it as a massage for your vagina and vulva, but from the inside. Read on for the mechanics of it all.

Let's start with endorphins. They are hormones produced and stored in the pituitary gland (see page 86) that act as neurotransmitters in the brain and throughout the nervous system. They whir around your synapses, creating feelings of happiness, joy, and even euphoria. Now, you're probably thinking, "How do I get hold of these?", right? Research has shown that exercise, eating chocolate, drinking wine, and getting massages all release endorphins. Know what else does? Orgasms!

Even aside from the rush of endorphins, the physical motion of orgasms on your clitoris and vagina tend to send you into good spasms. These little (or big!) clenches you can feel inside act like a highly specific massage, loosening up your muscles in a way that seems to help your uterus continue with its lining-shedding business more smoothly (see page 81).

Getting in the mood

Some folks are fully into heading downtown when they're on and feel extra horny to boot. Whether you're masturbating or enjoying period sex, be aware that you may need to do some extra prep or clean-up (see opposite for practical suggestions).

However, some people find it uncomfortable or painful to put pressure on their vulva and vagina during their period. Others literally faint at the sight of blood, making period sex impractical. Sex toys and erotic thoughts, images, and literature are great for when you aren't interested in a lot of touching but really want to get off. If touching elsewhere is okay, remember that you have other erogenous zones.

And if you're not feeling it or don't enjoy orgasms, you can still benefit from endorphins. Get outside for some vigorous exercise, book (or ask a friend or partner for) a massage, and settle down with a responsible amount of wine or chocolate.

Sexual healing

Endorphins allow your brain to reduce stress levels, provide pain relief, and create a natural high—isn't the human body incredible?

Can I have sex during my period?

If you and anyone you choose to be with is into period sex, enjoy! But it's not a rite of passage or an expectation, so if you're not eager, that's cool, too.

When it comes to period sex, remember that you should come first—literally and figuratively. Don't let anyone pressure you to have or not have sex on your period. If you have a partner who doesn't want to, do it yourself (see opposite). If your partner is eager for sexual activities but you're not interested, you have every right to say so. And no one should shame you for getting your period during sex or in their bed. If this happens, check that your partner wants to continue—consent is a dialogue.

The menstrual boudoir

When having sex on your period, there are a few practical considerations and extra preparations you may want to take on. Have a "sex blanket" or "period blanket" for catching bodily fluids and protecting your sheets and mattress—not because stains are embarrassing,

NOVEL REINVENTIONS
If you want all of the sex but none of the mess, menstrual cups have you covered.

There are a couple of menstrual cup designs that mimic the old-style diaphragm type of barrier birth control that was popular in the '60s and '70s. These cups are wider and flatter than the standard style and are worn very close to the cervix, so vaginal penetration is possible (and less messy).

but because postcoital laundry is a bit of a buzzkill. Layer up to save your free time for snuggles. A designated blanket made of fleece or another cozy and absorbent material works wonders underneath and isn't scratchy on your butt or face or knees (however you roll). Have a towel handy for a quick clean-up (so you don't leave bloody fingerprints on each other, the bedclothes, the doorknob, and so on). Most of all, have fun!

Practicalities
Your favorite fancy bedsheet soaking in the sink can turn fun times into household chores— but a designated blanket can be washed at your leisure!

Hormones

Hormones are what make the whole cycle happen. We haven't been taught nearly as much about this vital aspect of our bodies as we should have been. So here, in all their glory, are our hormones. In this chapter, we'll get the lowdown on them—where they come from, what they do, and how they can impact our health and well-being.

What are the hormones involved in the menstrual cycle?

There are a bunch of different hormones at play throughout the cycle, and every single one of them is key to keeping things moving.

First things first: a hormone is a chemical your body makes to jump-start functions in your body. When it comes to the menstrual cycle, the four hormones you need to know about are follicle-stimulating hormone (FSH), luteinizing hormone (LH), estrogen, and progesterone.

How the cycle works

Hormones are produced by glands, of which there are many in the body. Those involved in the reproductive system are known as the HPO axis. No, these are not characters in a new high-concept heist movie. HPO stands for the hypothalamus, the pituitary gland, and the ovaries. The hypothalamus, positioned in the middle of the brain, manages your core temperature, appetite, emotions, libido, and sleep cycles—it's like a personal assistant, therapist, erotic novel, and cozy cardigan in one. The pituitary gland hangs out right below the hypothalamus and controls puberty and growth. And the ovaries sit on either side of the uterus, where they produce egg cells (ova).

Your very first menstrual cycle kicks off when your hypothalamus releases a hormone called GnRH (gonadotropin-releasing hormone). GnRH stimulates the pituitary gland to start releasing FSH and LH. This causes egg-containing follicles (or egg sacs)

in the ovaries to mature, with one growing larger than the others. As the follicles mature, the cells around them develop and produce estrogen, which helps the uterine lining (or endometrium) grow. When estrogen levels get high enough, the pituitary gland releases a spike of LH, causing the largest follicle to release an egg: this is ovulation.

Now progesterone steps in. It causes structural changes in the uterine lining to prepare it for egg implantation and then pregnancy maintenance. If a fertilized egg implants (see page 113), the ovaries and, in particular, the ruptured follicle that previously contained the egg (the corpus luteum, to use its fancy name) continue to produce progesterone. This keeps the uterine lining

Your intricate system

There is a delicate balance between your hormones (like someone who can spin hula hoops on their hands, hips, and head) that's important for health.

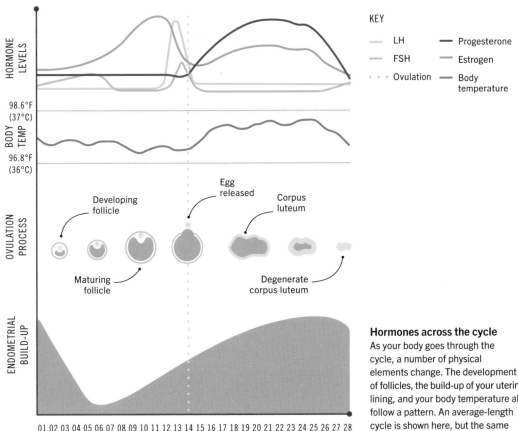

KEY

— LH	— Progesterone	
— FSH	— Estrogen	
· · · Ovulation	— Body temperature	

HORMONE LEVELS

98.6°F (37°C)

BODY TEMP

96.8°F (36°C)

OVULATION PROCESS

Egg released

Developing follicle

Corpus luteum

Maturing follicle

Degenerate corpus luteum

ENDOMETRIAL BUILD-UP

01 02 03 04 05 06 07 08 09 10 11 12 13 14 15 16 17 18 19 20 21 22 23 24 25 26 27 28

A 28-DAY MENSTRUAL CYCLE

Hormones across the cycle
As your body goes through the cycle, a number of physical elements change. The development of follicles, the build-up of your uterine lining, and your body temperature all follow a pattern. An average-length cycle is shown here, but the same stages take place in menstrual cycles of all lengths.

thick and the muscle of the uterus relaxed (so a fetus can fit inside it), as well as nurturing the fetus. If a fertilized egg doesn't implant, or the egg remains unfertilized, the corpus luteum shrivels up, and estrogen and progesterone levels drop, causing the uterine lining to shed—and voilà, there's your period! The first day of menstruation marks the beginning of the next cycle.

Rinse and repeat
It's important to be aware that, while this all happens regularly, it is probably a *different* regular for each person (see page 89). The "average" cycle may be 28 days long, but anywhere between 21 and 35 is totally fine, as long as it's fine for you. You should see your doctor if your cycle changes suddenly, as it's likely a sign that something else is amiss.

Why do some people start their periods really young and others not until later?

We don't know for sure what exactly makes each person start their period at a particular age, but there are a few factors that can nudge someone to either end of the range.

People usually experience menarche (their first period) anytime between the ages of 9 and 16. There is some evidence to suggest that menarchal age is inherited matrilineally—meaning members of a direct maternal line tend to begin menstruating at around the same age.

You'd be forgiven for thinking that, if someone's periods start early, they will end early, too, but that's not necessarily the case. Our menovulatory spans (see page 114) vary in length.

Starting outside the usual range

Early menarche (when a person's periods start before age 9) is a feature of precocious puberty (when puberty happens at a younger age than usual). Precocious puberty is rare and may have no apparent cause, but it is sometimes due to a tumor or genetic condition and can also be caused by cranial radiotherapy (a treatment for cancer) in childhood. It's possible to delay early periods by giving the child GnRH analogs, a drug that blocks the hormones that cause ovulation.

Even though 16 is the top of the normal range, if someone's period hasn't started by 14, then it's worth investigating. The sooner the cause is diagnosed, the easier it will be to address. It could be physiological or a chromosomal or hormonal condition (see page 93 for more on causes of menstrual irregularities). More research is needed on how environmental factors might impact or delay the onset of puberty.

"MENARCHE" IS GREEK AND PRONOUNCED LIKE THE WORD "ANARCHY"

Oh, and a missing menarche could be due to pregnancy—it's possible, though unlikely, to get pregnant before your first period. Because you ovulate before you menstruate, if you're sexually active at that time, you could be very unlucky and get pregnant in your first cycle.

Why is my cycle a different length from my friend's?

Each of us bleeds to the rhythm of our own drum, so to speak. Everyone's hormones are slightly different, and our unique systems each find a balance of their own.

To understand how menstrual cycle length varies, we need to look at its two phases.

The phase before ovulation is known as the follicular phase, during which eggs develop in follicles (egg sacs) in an ovary, preparing for ovulation (see page 86). For one person, this bit of the cycle could regularly be only 7 days—while, for someone else, it might last for 21 days. It's not known why this variation occurs. Periods themselves average 2–7 days.

After ovulation comes the luteal phase, during which the uterus gears up for a pregnancy or a period. This is pretty reliably 14–15 days long for most people, meaning it's possible to work out when you ovulated by counting back from the day you got your period. In rare cases, the luteal phase can be shorter or longer than this.

So in a group of menstruators, each person's cycle length could be different. And, as discussed on page 25, we don't synchronize.

Know your body

Cycles tend to settle into a reliable pattern after the first few years of menstruating, but if yours haven't, see a doctor. You can also seek medical advice if your cycle is very long and affecting your attempts to conceive, or so short that it feels as though you're constantly on. You can chart your cycle (see pages 90–91) to discover your cycle length.

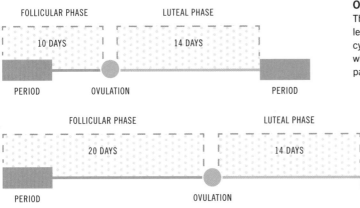

FOLLICULAR PHASE | LUTEAL PHASE

10 DAYS | 14 DAYS

PERIOD | OVULATION | PERIOD

FOLLICULAR PHASE | LUTEAL PHASE

20 DAYS | 14 DAYS

PERIOD | OVULATION | PERIOD

Overall cycle lengths
The variation in follicular phase length explains why some people's cycles last for as few as 21 days, while others' last for up to 35 (see page 87 for an average cycle).

What's the best way to track my cycle?

Charting your cycle is a surprisingly simple way to learn about your body. Whether you prefer using apps or traditional calendars, track with curiosity, not expectations.

Cycle charting or tracking allows you to gain knowledge about how your menstrual cycle works, so you can observe and even predict the timing of events like ovulation and recognize any signs that something might be wrong.

You can track your cycle generally or for a specific purpose. For instance, you might want to plot your personal bests in sports training on your chart or assess your cycle for evidence of a medical condition such as PMDD (see page 99). It's very handy to be able to whip out a record of your last 12 cycles and reel it off to your doctor to show you know your stuff.

Start tracking

There are a couple of ways to track your cycle. The low-tech way is to use your normal diary, planner, phone calendar, wall calendar, a spreadsheet, or even draw your own cute chart and make notes during your cycle at the level of detail you want (more on that in a moment).

Alternatively, you could use one of the many apps available, which simplify the process by allowing you to toggle settings to track different aspects of your cycle. Ignore the ones run by tampon companies and the like, though— they're just thinly veiled ads and will bombard you with branding. There are some excellent independent apps out there, but as with all apps, check you know what they're doing with your data. Some are transparent about the

Knowledge is power

Understanding the workings of your menstrual cycle gives you a sense of physical self-knowledge that is deeply reassuring and empowering.

data going toward menstrual research, while others sell to marketers who could use the data to track your purchasing choices or tailor advertising to you at specific points in your cycle. Do your homework when selecting.

What to track

What you should track depends on what you want to get out of the process:
⬥ **If you're** starting out, focus on period length, amount of blood, and cycle length to see if you're within the average ranges (2–7 days per period, 21–35 days per cycle). Once it's part of your routine, level up by adding in productivity, exercise, and mood each day. You may also want to roughly establish when you're ovulating (see the chart on page 87) and how long your follicular phase lasts (see page 89).

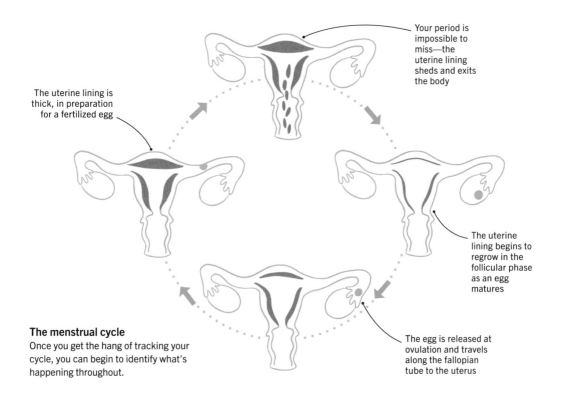

The uterine lining is thick, in preparation for a fertilized egg

Your period is impossible to miss—the uterine lining sheds and exits the body

The uterine lining begins to regrow in the follicular phase as an egg matures

The egg is released at ovulation and travels along the fallopian tube to the uterus

The menstrual cycle
Once you get the hang of tracking your cycle, you can begin to identify what's happening throughout.

💧 **If you** suspect a medical issue, such as PMDD (see page 99), endometriosis (page 106), or PCOS (see page 107), track the previous plus pain, energy levels, and sleep patterns.

💧 **If you're** using the Fertility Awareness Method (see page 129) either to get pregnant or to prevent pregnancy, you'll want to know when you're in your fertile window (see page 113) so you can have or avoid unprotected sex accordingly. Note your morning temperature each day (see the chart on page 87), along with descriptions of the texture of your cervical mucus (see page 112), your energy levels, and your sense of smell, which may be heightened during your fertile window. Also note when you have unprotected sex.

💧 **If you** think you might be perimenopausal, track sleep patterns, length of period and cycle, and heavy or light days to see if the pattern is changing (see pages 146–147).

💧 **If it's** all about sports, synchronize a fitness device or smartwatch that tracks your stats with your cycle—many now include a built-in cycle-charting feature.

I love charting my cycle. I had no clue how my period worked before I started charting, but within a year, I was a highly politicized menstrual activist—so, you know, you do the math! It is period positive to find out about yourself—especially a part of yourself that was once considered taboo.

"Periods are a vital sign—
charting your cycle tells you
a lot about your health."

What causes irregular cycles?

Your body is a delicately balanced system—if something's thrown out of whack, you may see the effects in your menstrual cycle.

Cycles should settle down into regular patterns within a couple of years after menarche and about three months after coming off the pill. It's not uncommon to experience irregular cycles at one time or another, though, if your HPO axis (see page 86) becomes disrupted.

Potential disruptors

Stress can wreak havoc with your hormones. It can stop the hypothalamus from producing GnRH, which means the pituitary gland doesn't produce FSH and LH, so you don't ovulate. This may be your body protecting you from a pregnancy it senses you can't handle by pressing pause on periods (a nonessential bodily function).

Extreme changes to your diet and exercise regimen can also affect menstruation, as changes to your metabolism can trigger the hypothalamus to shut down menstruation. Periods usually begin again when things return to normal, but keep your doctor informed either way.

On rare occasions, it's not your cycle that's disrupted, but the bleeding itself. FGM procedures or scarring and rare congenital conditions affecting the vaginal opening can cause hematocolpos—when menstrual blood collects in the vagina but has no route, or too small a passageway, to flow out. There are specialists who can address this sensitively.

It is possible to have irregular cycles with no specific cause. It's always worth investigating, so push your doctor to look into it further.

Irregularity factors	
Illness	Being unwell can cause your HPO axis to cease normal operation
Diet	Calorific and nutritional changes that affect metabolism can stop menstruation
Exercise	Intense training regimes (such as those of pro athletes) affect metabolism
Stress	Both psychological and physiological stress can affect the normal pattern of the HPO axis
Weight fluctuation	Sudden weight gain or loss can affect your cycle by impairing ovulation
Medication	Generally, medication containing steroids can affect the pituitary gland or ovaries, and stop ovulation

How do my hormones affect my mood?

The hormones involved in the menstrual cycle also have a rhythmical impact on your mood. Knowing when the "up" and "down" times are can help you feel more in control.

As we know, hormones control the menstrual cycle. The same hormones that trigger ovulation and menstruation in each repetition of your cycle also impact your mood—as you've probably noticed, when you're feeling bad.

You may not have linked these hormones to the positive effects they can have, though. There are predictable patterns of how your mood can lift, as well as dip, based on where you are in your cycle.

Undulations of mood

The cycle starts with your period—you may feel the need to hunker down, withdraw, or even just sleep. Feeling exhausted is pretty common, particularly during the first couple of days of bleeding. This can be due to the stress of managing your period, feeling tired as your uterus works overtime, or even having less iron than usual, if you have a heavy flow.

Once your period is over, for the remainder of the follicular phase (see page 89), estrogen keeps you pretty peppy. It has a positive impact on energy levels and alertness. Right before ovulation, you may feel especially confident, creative, and sexy.

After you ovulate and hit the luteal phase, though, progesterone takes over. As levels rise, you can be slammed with low mood; anger; low confidence; and, my least favorite, paranoia. That's right, you guessed it—it's PMS.

Premenstrual syndrome is the name given to a collection of physical and emotional symptoms (see page 98) that can begin up to 10 days

Down times
Many people feel low, drained, and irritable in the days leading up to and during their period.

that are genuinely annoying. There are a few compelling studies by respected researchers showing that menstruators who lived with people who understood what they were going through reported fewer symptoms. It seems that trying to please a partner or mask symptoms in front of them can reduce your threshold for tolerating irritation.

Understanding how different moods correlate with each part of your cycle can help you feel less overwhelmed by challenging emotions and sensations when you notice them. But make sure you pay attention to external factors that can affect your mood as well.

before the bleeding phase of a typical menstrual cycle, as progesterone levels rise. Mood changes are not always just down to hormones, though. They may also come from reacting to the physical symptoms—many people try to ignore them or hide them from others, leading to increased irritability.

Premenstrual symptoms tend to recede once your period starts. After that, you swing back around to the next follicular phase, and so on.

It's all about perspective

Interestingly, there may be even more going on than the above. At "happy" phases in your cycle, you may not be as tuned into things

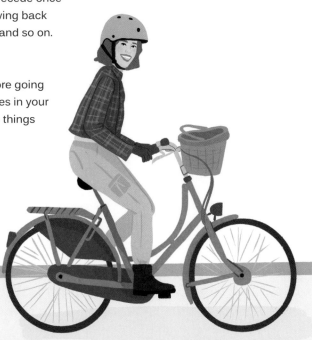

Up times
Once your period's over, you may feel happier, more energized, and ready to take on the world.

Are certain stages of the cycle best for certain activities?

We know that different parts of the cycle can bring on various feelings, but how can we use that knowledge? Read on to find out how to get the most out of every stage.

The thing to remember about the hormones that govern the menstrual cycle is that they work to a cyclical rhythm. This means, as we've seen on pages 94–95, that there are predictable patterns in the effects they have on your mood as they gear you up for getting busy or getting bloody.

Everyone is different, but many people find they're better at certain activities during particular parts of their cycle, compared to other times. You might be experiencing varying moods without even realizing. Identifying them enables you to adjust your daily activities accordingly and form a deeper relationship with your cycle. Try aligning your plans as suggested opposite for a few months and see if you feel more in tune with your cycle.

Find your flow
See if you can harness the energetic phase of your cycle for new projects, and enjoy the flow state that may come more naturally at this time.

Harnessing your energy

During the follicular phase of your cycle (see page 89), you'll likely have a good amount of creative energy, thanks to high levels of estrogen. You can focus your mind on projects. You may feel more motivated and productive and be more alert to your surroundings. You may also feel more confident and resourceful.

It's easy to accidentally overcommit during this phase, so watch out for a tendency to stay out late one night too many or buy yet another succulent plant .... You may also notice that you find more people attractive around this time or feel more engaged in romantic relationships. You might feel super horny and want to masturbate more often than during the rest of the month, or find that you are feeling particularly amorous toward a partner.

Slowing down

Once you ovulate, your body is no longer looking for someone to make a baby with. As the primordial procreation urge disappears, it can drag your mood down with it. Even if you didn't want to get pregnant, you may still have a feeling of "missed opportunity" that you can't quite put your finger on. This can feel unsettling, but it is easier to navigate if you know it's coming. During the luteal phase, the rise in progesterone means your fuse is likely to be shorter, which means you may judge yourself and others a bit more quickly and harshly than usual.

ENJOY THE DOWN TIMES. GET COZY, REST, AND STORE UP SOME ENERGY.

These feelings are real—you should never be made to feel like they're "just down to hormones" and don't matter. In fact, look to see whether there's a grain of truth to any of your judgments during this time. You're likely to be more tuned into annoyances, problems, and untrustworthy people now than at other times in your cycle.

As your luteal phase continues and you eventually reach your period, you may start to feel more and more flat. If possible, embrace the flatness, rather than resisting it. Take time out if you can. Make a blanket fort and hunker down. Use orgasms to ease cramps (see page 82). Keep exercising and eating healthily, but take activities at a gentler pace if you need to.

It's not just pain from cramps or constipation (see page 98) that can make you want to curl up in a ball during the first couple of days of your cycle, it's also a general sensation of the blahs. So go easy on yourself before your next follicular phase—after all, it's right around the corner.

Live in tune

Try making plans according to your body's rhythm. Align activities with how you feel—physically, emotionally, and psychologically—in the different stages of your cycle.

What is PMS and what's the best way to manage it?

Well, I can tell you the worst way: by pretending it's not happening. Acknowledging all parts of your cycle—including the less fun bits—will allow you to find ways to manage them.

Premenstrual tension (or premenstrual syndrome) refers to symptoms that appear in the couple of weeks before menstruation. You might experience cramps; bloating; constipation; acne; sore boobs; low mood; junk-food cravings; anxiety; and, often hardest to pin down, a feeling that everyone is out to get you.

Diet and exercise

Some symptoms are reduced by eating well, so try to avoid giving in to the comfort food and salt cravings caused by hormone fluctuations. Candy, chips, and other processed foods might make you feel better in the moment but won't help your digestion, bowels, skin, energy levels, or water retention (see page 79).

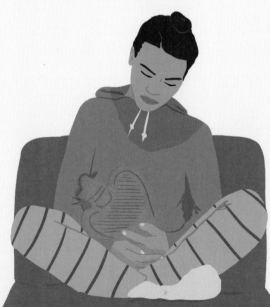

High progesterone levels prior to your period can slow digestion, making you constipated. Eat fruit or fiber every morning and get ready for the period poop. Yes, it's a thing—many people experience constipation during their period.

Exercise is another great remedy. Stretches, core strengthening, dancing, or a brisk walk will get your blood pumping, improve your mood, and ease cramps (see page 79). You can also soothe cramps with safe use of a hot water bottle, heating pad, or microwavable bean bag.

Other strategies

If your PMS is hard to manage, speak to a doctor. Hormonal contraception can help (see page 120), as can pain or stress management techniques, and/orsupplements (try vitamin B6, magnesium, and calcium—though first confirm with your doctor that these won't interfere with other conditions or medications). Mostly though, go easy on yourself and talk to others about how you feel.

Changing the way you think about PMS (and your cycle as a whole) might also help. People gave it a name because it's seen as a negative part of the cycle—but it's worth remembering that PMS is simply a collection of cues that your period is around the corner. The cues don't all have to be seen as negative.

How do I know if I have PMDD?

If PMS is ruining your day, week, or relationships, it could be premenstrual dysphoric disorder—poor mental health that occurs before and during your period.

PMDD is severe low mood that coincides with the premenstrual and menstrual phases of your cycle. A number of possible causes have been suggested, including interaction between estrogen and the brain chemical serotonin earlier in the cycle, genetics, immune factors, and the effects of past trauma. This is a treatable medical condition—you shouldn't have to suffer.

The threshold for diagnosing PMDD is usually "if it's disrupting your life"—so it's pretty subjective. It should be clear to you that something's wrong with your mental health and that it's linked to your cycle, predictably going away during or just after your period.

What you can do

You can alleviate some aspects of PMDD by eating healthily and getting plenty of sleep, water, and exercise during the luteal phase (see page 89), but these things can only go so far. Your doctor might recommend antidepressants, hormonal contraceptives, GnRH analogs with HRT (see page 148), or psychotherapy.

As with everything menstrual, more research into PMDD is desperately needed. Recent studies indicate that many sufferers may have been misdiagnosed with bipolar disorder, because there is some overlap in reported symptoms. It's known that PMDD can worsen with age and that people who experience it may also be prone to postpartum depression.

If you don't realize you have PMDD, it's likely you think it's run-of-the-mill PMS. And because of period taboos and tacky jokes about grumpy menstruators being "on the rag," you might feel your PMDD is just something you have to tolerate. Even worse, you might believe that everyone else around you feels just as bad as you, but they're somehow controlling themselves, so why can't you?

That is not true. You don't have to tolerate it, and no one should dismiss your concerns. Ignore anyone trying to convince you it's "just hormones," or to "suck it up." Start tracking your symptoms against your cycle (see pages 90–91) in a PMDD diary and take it to a specialist.

How can I use synthetic hormones to regulate my periods?

If aspects of your periods—such as pain, flow, or cycle length—are interfering with your life, you may consider using hormonal birth control to manage the symptoms.

Synthetic hormones are chemicals that mimic the actions of the ones our bodies produce. Hormonal contraception contains synthetic versions of estrogen and progesterone (see page 86). Taking these hormones in prescribed doses can override the natural patterns of the menstrual cycle, which means they can help your body regulate some of the harder-to-manage symptoms of your period.

Managing problematic symptoms

For people struggling with cycle length, heavy flow, pain, or irregular cycles, the combined pill (see pages 120–121) is commonly prescribed. When on the pill, you don't have a "real" period but instead have a withdrawal bleed (see page 122). This tends to be lighter and shorter than a normal period, and regular, since your system contains exactly the same hormone levels each month. What's more, with your hormones on an even keel, you'll likely see improvements in other areas, such as mood and skin. The pill has some common side effects that you should know about (see pages 126–127). The implant and the IUD (see pages 124–125) are alternatives; speak to a doctor to determine which would be best for you.

A gentle observation: if you only want to use birth control to stop periods because you think they're gross or inconvenient, consider revising your relationship with menstrual blood (see page 47). Also weigh up whether the convenience is worth the side effects or cost (see pages 126–127).

Reasons for a prescription
As well as preventing pregnancy, hormonal birth control can help with a number of symptoms.

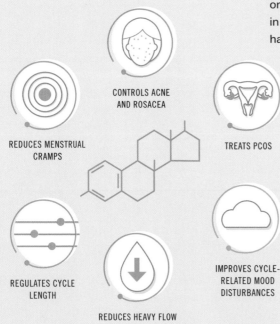

CONTROLS ACNE AND ROSACEA

REDUCES MENSTRUAL CRAMPS

TREATS PCOS

REGULATES CYCLE LENGTH

IMPROVES CYCLE-RELATED MOOD DISTURBANCES

REDUCES HEAVY FLOW

What happens to your period if you're trans?

It can be tough to navigate menstruation at all stages of your transition, but there are things you can do to make it easier.

For many trans men and nonbinary folks, periods can raise issues, particularly for those who are yet to, or don't intend to, transition hormonally. Menstrual cycles can impact how you feel about your gender identity. You may have some visceral reactions to menstrual taboos if you've internalized them or to blood and bleeding in a process our culture associates with binary gender in general, and with "becoming a woman" in particular. There are also added issues of having to navigate periods in public as a gender-nonconforming person who menstruates, as well as the choices you make about how you personally manage your periods.

You may worry about being "outed" by PMS symptoms, leaks, or products. It's tough to navigate periods in a positive way if you don't want to have or talk about them, and society doesn't help. Dialogues initiated by trans activists and researchers are increasingly available, and change is happening, but periods, bathrooms, and "who menstruates" are all too often a baseless and discriminatory touchpoint for transphobes.

Feeling more comfortable

There are practical ways to queer your menstrual milieu. Look at influencing your built environment: for instance, if you live, work, or study somewhere with communal bathrooms, ask for a trash can to be placed in the men's room.

You can change your language, too—adopt a gender-neutral term that asserts your right to have periods, such as "menstruator" or "person with periods." (A friend of mine calls their period a "wolfcycle.")

Before and after transitioning

Not everyone chooses—or has access to—gender-affirming hormone therapy. If you do transition hormonally, though, the changes you'll experience will affect your cycle.

In the first few months of taking testosterone, your periods might become lighter and shorter and arrive later, though some people experience heavier or longer-lasting periods for a few cycles. In all cases, after a while, they will stop completely. It's important to report any spotting, as this can signal that you are metabolizing testosterone particularly quickly, which means you'll need a higher dose so your periods don't come back.

Even after hormonal transition, ensure you still get and respond to letters offering screenings for cervical and breast cancer (which is still a risk even after top surgery).

Get support

There's a growing array of resources for trans and nonbinary menstruators and reputable organizations that can help you navigate finding inclusive gynecologists.

Why is my skin so bad during my period and around ovulation?

It's common to experience hormonal acne at certain times in your cycle. It happens for most people at some point, but there are ways to deal with it.

Acne can occur at any age and is often a normal part of a healthy menstrual cycle, caused by hormonal fluctuations. In particular, high testosterone levels and/or high sensitivity to testosterone can lead to breakouts around ovulation and during your period.

Increased testosterone is related to acne, excess hair growth, and a tendency to sweat. All your skin glands—sebaceous glands, oil glands, and hair follicles—contain testosterone receptors, which is why this hormone affects your skin. The chin and forehead are the places most susceptible to hormonal acne, along with the upper body, chest, and back.

What to do

Sometimes a good cleansing regimen is all that's needed for hormonal acne to clear up on its own. You can also try topical creams. If your acne is impacting your self-worth or mood, see a dermatologist or endocrinologist about prescription acne meds or suppressing testosterone production by taking the pill or testosterone reception blockers. Even if you get rid of acne once, though, it can come back like clockwork during your next cycle.

Keep in mind that perfect skin is a myth. Good hydration, sun protection, and a regular cleansing routine will usually stop the worst breakouts—but don't let anyone make you feel at fault if you still have acne or acne scars despite all of this.

Self-care

Don't stop at a skin-care regimen if your skin flares up. Ensure that you also get plenty of sleep and eat fresh vegetables—and embrace your face!

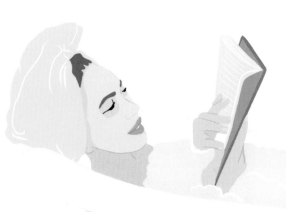

Why am I so horny about halfway through my cycle?

You might have noticed that you feel especially in the mood for sex at certain points in your cycle—there's a reason for this.

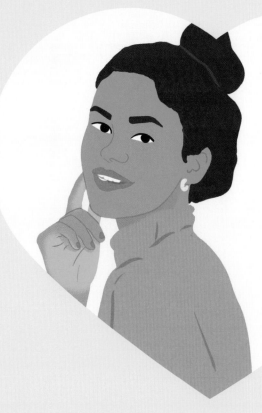

One of the many things affected by the hormonal fluctuations throughout your menstrual cycle is your desire to have sex. Libido, or sex drive, changes throughout, but it commonly peaks around ovulation, which tends to be around the midpoint—though it may be that you ovulate earlier or later in your cycle (see page 89).

This increase in horniness just before ovulation happens as your body tries to encourage you to introduce it to some sperm. In basic terms, your body is trying to make the most of your fertile window to create more people.

Ebb and flow

The amount of sex you want to have at any given time isn't always simply down to your hormone levels. Sexual desire is a spectrum from asexual (where you don't experience sexual desire) to allosexual (where you do), and we don't always sit at the same point along it. Fluctuating hormones might explain some of the regular patterns you notice, though.

You may find it desirable to have different types of sexual and nonsexual contact and comfort at different times of the month.

You may also find that you feel less like having sex just before and during your period, when estrogen levels are low. But everyone's different—there are no hard-and-fast rules about how hard and fast you choose to get.

Oh, and while we're on the subject, did I mention that orgasms can help ease menstrual cramps? It's like a little massage for your vagina from within (see page 82 for more).

Is my immune system affected by my cycle?

Recent research and anecdotal evidence point to a link between the menstrual cycle and the immune system, but there's lots we still don't know.

Your immune system works to protect your body from harmful intruders, such as viruses and irritants. But what does that have to do with periods? It involves hormones—what's still not clear is exactly how the connection works.

There is evidence to suggest that fluctuation of both estrogen and progesterone levels can have an effect on the immune system. Some research indicates that the higher levels of estrogen during the follicular phase of the cycle (see page 89) might cause a heightened immune response, meaning you're less likely to be ill. Then, once ovulation has happened and estrogen levels drop, the immune system seems to step back. It's also been suggested that rising levels of progesterone in the luteal phase add to this effect—some people are more susceptible to sickness during this time, so experience more minor ailments when their period rolls around.

An increased immune response is great for fighting infection, but if it goes into overdrive, it can impact autoimmune illnesses and chronic conditions such as diabetes and asthma. Some people with these conditions have reported worse symptoms before and during their periods. Studies also indicate that inflammation—one of the immune system's defense mechanisms—worsens cramps.

Why the link?

Biologically speaking, a heightened immune response helps you stay healthy so you can make a baby (which is what the ovaries are up for, even if you're not). This might explain why the immune system seems to be stronger in the follicular phase.

And what about when immunity seems to decrease? One suggestion is that your body limits your immune response to help any sperm in the genital tract to survive, increasing the chance of conception. Or the dip might be to reduce the chance of your immune system rejecting a fertilized egg (half of which, technically, counts as a foreign body).

The jury is still out on this one. Thankfully, researchers are eager to look into the question further, so there may be answers in the future.

Advances in understanding

The more we learn about periods, the more we realize how much we don't know. Increasingly, institutions are able to get funding for menstrual studies.

"Keep up to date with reports from reputable sources—you deserve to know the facts."

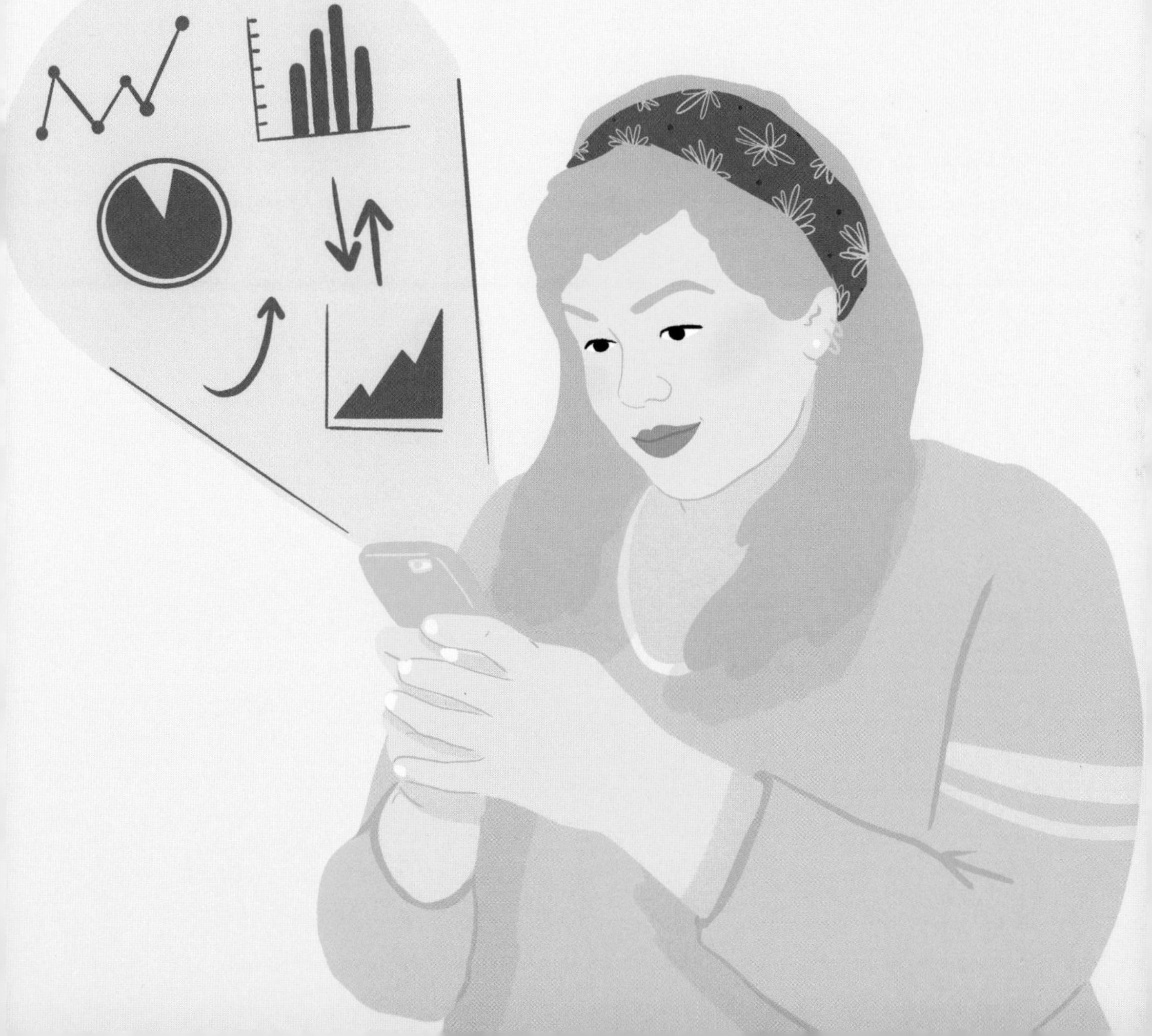

What is endometriosis?

With painful symptoms and an average of eight years to reach a diagnosis, having endometriosis can be an incredibly frustrating experience—but medics are beginning to listen.

Endometriosis occurs when the tissue that normally forms the uterine lining (the endometrium) also grows outside the uterus, in the surrounding areas. In the luteal phase (see page 89), when the lining thickens, so does the rogue tissue. Then, during menstruation, this tissue bleeds inside the body. Typical symptoms are pelvic pain, extreme cramps, and painful sex.

Getting a diagnosis

Endometrial tissue growing on the ovaries can be diagnosed via sonogram. Otherwise, an exploratory keyhole surgery is needed to see where the tissue is growing.

Endometriosis gradually worsens, and, if left untreated, can cause scarring that blocks the fallopian tubes, leading to infertility. Tubal blockage may be screened for with an x-ray.

For people whose illness is slow to develop or those with lighter periods, anti-inflammatories can help with pain. But in most cases, medical or surgical treatment is required. Medical treatments include the combined pill (see pages 120–121) or a hormone blocker, both of which suppress tissue growth. Surgical treatment involves removal of endometrial tissue under general anesthetic; it may need to be repeated. Ultimately, you may opt for a hysterectomy. (Be aware that this will trigger menopause—see page 143.)

Increasing awareness

So how common is endometriosis? It's hard to tell, as diagnosis is slow. The condition is underresearched and often dismissed as bad cramps—many family doctors haven't had enough training on what to look for. Sometimes symptoms go unnoticed or are attributed to something else. If you have no luck, change doctors and keep asking. You are not alone.

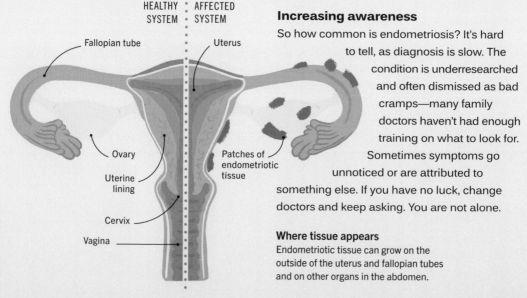

HEALTHY SYSTEM : AFFECTED SYSTEM

Fallopian tube

Uterus

Ovary

Patches of endometriotic tissue

Uterine lining

Cervix

Vagina

Where tissue appears
Endometriotic tissue can grow on the outside of the uterus and fallopian tubes and on other organs in the abdomen.

What is PCOS?

Polycystic ovary syndrome (PCOS) is a fairly common hormonal condition that can be managed.

PCOS is associated with abnormal hormone levels, including high testosterone. The condition affects the ovaries, the follicles (egg sacs) within which stop developing at a certain point in each cycle. The name "polycystic" comes from the follicles' resemblance to cysts (small, fluid-filled lumps). While these follicles can still contain eggs, disruption to the HPO axis (see page 86) means that some people with PCOS don't ovulate regularly, leading to irregular or absent periods.

The other symptoms of PCOS include difficulty conceiving, thinning head hair, acne, extra hair on the face and/or body, and a tendency to be thicker around the middle.

Researchers have found some links between PCOS and type 2 diabetes, high cholesterol, heart disease, and endometrial cancer.

There's a lot we still don't know about what causes PCOS.

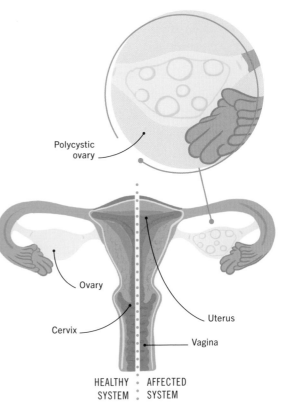

Polycystic ovary

Ovary

Cervix

Uterus

Vagina

HEALTHY SYSTEM · AFFECTED SYSTEM

Affected ovaries
During each menstrual cycle, follicles in the ovaries grow to up to ⅜in (9mm) in size, causing the ovaries to become enlarged.

Diagnosis and treatment

You can be diagnosed if you have two out of three features—polycystic ovaries (seen on an sonogram), infrequent or absent periods, and high levels of testosterone or excess hair growth and acne. Doctors rarely diagnose young people or new menstruators with PCOS, preferring to wait for cycles to settle into regularity. If you feel like something is wrong, though, don't be afraid to push for further investigation sooner.

There is no overall treatment available for PCOS. Each symptom is treated separately—for instance, fertility issues can be addressed (see pages 118–19), and there are medications to combat unwanted hair growth.

IN THE UK, **1 IN 10** PEOPLE WITH OVARIES ARE **AFFECTED BY PCOS**

What are the symptoms of gynecological cancers?

Womb-related cancers are underresearched and underdiagnosed and don't always have obvious symptoms, so it's vital to be aware of the early signs.

I'm so glad you're reading this—not to be melodramatic, but it could literally save your life. As with other forms of cancer, survival rates for gynecological cancers are much lower for those with late diagnoses. It won't pay to take a "wait and see" approach.

Be aware of the symptoms and check your vulva and vagina regularly to feel for anything unusual, in the same way you would check your breasts for lumps. If you notice changes, see a doctor. In cases of ovarian cancer, the symptoms usually take a while to show up. With the exception of cervical cancer, which is more common in younger people, the risk of getting these cancers increases with age. Trans guys should be aware of the symptoms, too.

Speak up if you're concerned

Studies show that people are sometimes afraid to report symptoms because they don't like using words like "vagina" and "discharge." Practice the sentences you will say to the doctor at home, then get that visit booked. Spread the word— taboos shouldn't stop people from getting help.

Signs to watch out for

The symptoms below are listed in order of frequency, from most to least common.

Common symptoms	Endometrial cancer	Ovarian cancer	Cervical cancer	Vulval cancer	Vaginal cancer
	⬦ Post-menopausal bleeding	⬦ Increased abdominal size and persistent bloating	⬦ Bleeding between periods	⬦ Lasting itch	⬦ Bleeding between periods
	⬦ Bleeding between periods	⬦ Persistent pelvic/ abdominal pain	⬦ Bleeding after sex	⬦ Pain and soreness	⬦ Post-menopausal bleeding
	⬦ Very heavy periods	⬦ Change in bowel habits	⬦ Painful sex	⬦ Thickened, raised, discolored patches of skin	⬦ Bleeding after sex
	⬦ Unusual discharge	⬦ Difficulty eating or nausea	⬦ Unusual vaginal discharge	⬦ An open sore or growth	⬦ Painful sex
		⬦ Increased urinary frequency		⬦ A mole that changes shape or color	⬦ Unusual discharge
				⬦ A lump or swelling	⬦ A lump
					⬦ Lasting itch
					⬦ Painful urination
					⬦ Persistent pain

What is the HPV shot for?

Our response to human papilloma virus (HPV), a common STI, provides a great example of a successful public health campaign.

HPV is a sexually transmitted infection (STI) that is responsible for 99.7 percent of cases of cervical cancer. HPV is very common, has no symptoms, and is easy to transmit during unprotected sex, so it's important to understand the risks. It can cause cancer of the cervix, anus, or genitals; throat cancer; and genital warts.

Thankfully, there is a vaccine, which you may have had already—starting in 2006, an HPV shot has been available and is now recommended for all genders from adolescence.

Not everyone has been or can be vaccinated. Even if you weren't vaccinated as a teen, you can get the shot in adulthood via your doctor, pharmacies, and nonprofit organizations such as Planned Parenthood.

Getting a Pap smear

Another way HPV is addressed is through Pap smears and HPV tests. This quick procedure is normally done at your doctor's office or clinic. If you're 21–29, a Pap test is recommended every 3 years, plus an HPV test every 5 years, or both, if you're 30–65. A clinician will swab your cervix and test for signs of HPV and abnormal cells. The test can be stressful, and stress makes the vagina tighten, so it may cause discomfort at the time, but your clinician will be swift and professional.

If you have experienced trauma or sexual assault, you may ask to have your screening with specialist trauma protocols in place. If you are trans or nonbinary, you can ask for extra support or an inclusive provider to make your appointment less stressful, if needed.

THE HPV SHOT IS

EFFECTIVE

AGAINST THE TWO MOST HIGH-RISK TYPES OF HPV, WHICH CAUSE **80%** OF ALL KNOWN **CERVICAL CANCERS**

What might happen next

If any abnormal cells are spotted, you'll be called in for a procedure called a colposcopy, so that a specialist can examine a tiny section of your cervix where the abnormal cells were found. Further follow-up will depend on the results of this procedure.

Essential self-care

Cervical screenings and vaccinations are huge advances in catching cancer early and could actually save your life.

Fertility and contraception

We can't talk about menstrual cycles without a deep dive into the reason we have them: fertility. Whatever your choices around conception and contraception, understanding the practical details of it all is valuable—from signs of ovulation to signs of pregnancy, and everything in between.

How do I know when I'm most likely to conceive?

Your body may provide clues that help identify your fertile window (the time when you're most likely to get pregnant), but without medical intervention, you can't know for sure.

Nothing is guaranteed without a blood or urine test, but there are *lots* of physical signs of ovulation.

Signs to look out for

As you chart your cycle (see pages 90–91), look for the following signs:

◗ **A rise** in temperature. Your temperature runs slightly higher during the second half of your cycle (see the chart on page 87). When it first rises at the midpoint of your cycle (look for a rise of 0.4–0.9°F [0.2–0.5°C]), you're likely to be in your fertile window.

◗ **Slippery cervical** mucus (a secretion from the cervix). The consistency of cervical mucus changes throughout your cycle. When you're about to ovulate, it becomes more slippery and wet (like semen or egg white in texture) and passes the stretch test (see below). You can track it simply by checking the toilet paper after you first pee every day.

◗ **Mittelschmerz**—a little twinge in the ovary that some people can feel as the follicle ruptures to release an egg.

◗ **Increased energy** levels.

◗ **Bloating**.

◗ **Breast tenderness**.

◗ **Increased libido**.

◗ **A stronger** sense of smell, or just heightened senses generally.

◗ **A change** in the position of your cervix. Get used to checking it by feeling it with a finger to track its position. Low and wet? Ovulating! High and dry? Not ovulating!

There are apps available (period trackers and fertility apps) that can help you gather data on many of these signs. You can also seek out workshops dedicated to learning how to spot the signs (see page 129).

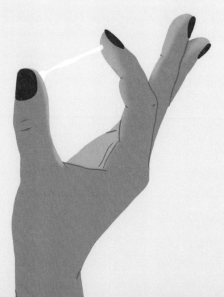

Cervical mucus stretch test
Press your index and middle fingers together and coat them in your cervical mucus. Now separate them by a few centimeters. If the mucus stretches in a line between them without breaking, it's likely you are in your fertile window.

How does conception happen?

There are so many factors at work in conception that it's amazing it ever happens at all. Statistically, it's cool you're alive to read this!

It surprised me when I found out conception usually takes place in the fallopian tube, not the uterus. So the egg doesn't have far to go before the sperm finds it, whereas the sperm has to travel farther than you may have thought.

Conditions have to be just right for conception. During the fertile window (a few days leading up to and hours following the ovulation of a healthy, mature egg), cervical mucus becomes slippery and easy for sperm to swim through. Several brands of fertility lubricant are designed to mimic the texture of fertile mucus and enhance the quality and quantity of the stuff that the cervix provides.

You also need to bank on the quality and quantity of that sperm, in terms of motility (how well they are able to travel in the right direction) and sperm count. A normal sperm count is, at the low end, 15 million per milliliter of semen.

Conception

If things are going swimmingly, the sperm can get to your uterus and up into your fallopian tubes. If these are blocked for any reason, such as advanced endometriosis (see page 106) or internal scarring caused by pelvic infections, conception can't happen unless the issue is addressed surgically.

Now, either the sperm needs to hang out in your fallopian tube for a few days (up to five or so), waiting for the egg to be released, or, if it's within 12 hours of ovulation (an easy window to miss), the egg and the sperm might combine right away. *Might*.

Once fertilized, the egg should make its way along the fallopian tube to the uterus, developing as it goes (see page 125 for a note on ectopic pregnancies). This journey takes roughly five days—implantation generally happens on day five after conception.

Implantation

When the fertilized egg arrives at the uterus, the uterine lining must be suitably thick (ideally, at least 7mm) for implantation to be successful. If conditions are right, the fertilized egg might burrow into the uterine lining. *Might*.

And that's conception. Pretty amazing, right?

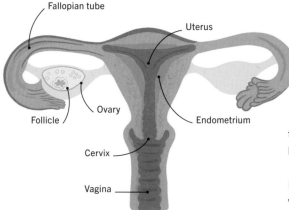

Labels: Fallopian tube, Uterus, Ovary, Follicle, Endometrium, Cervix, Vagina

Where the action takes place
An ovary releases an egg into the fallopian tube. The egg travels toward the uterus. If it is fertilized on the way, it may then implant into the lining of the uterus, and pregnancy may begin.

What is my "biological clock"?

We've talked about the fertile window in each menstrual cycle (see page 112), but there's also a fertile window within your lifetime during which you are able to become pregnant.

Back when marriage and two-point-four children seemed to be on the agenda of cultural expectations, "your biological clock is ticking" was a creeptastic jibe used to panic people into settling down and getting pregnant naturally before their egg reserves diminished. This is 100 percent gross—but a tiny bit realistic.

The ovaries start out with all of the egg cells they'll ever produce before you're even born, so you have a finite supply of viable eggs. The "ticking" of the "biological clock" refers to the countdown to the end of the menovulatory span, as your egg reserves are depleted.

Generally speaking, fertility starts to wane from your mid-thirties, but at this stage, this usually means an increase in the number of cycles it takes to become pregnant, not an end to your fertility, full stop. Fertility doesn't end entirely until menopause (see page 142), but egg quality and quantity begin to decrease in the mid-thirties and more rapidly so after 40, making it harder to become pregnant or maintain a healthy pregnancy. So if you're planning to conceive naturally, you should bear this in mind so you can make the right choices for yourself.

Your menovulatory span

The word "menovulatory" merges "menstruation" and "ovulation." Your menovulatory span is the phase of your lifetime in which you ovulate and menstruate.

Freezing eggs

Some people wonder if they should freeze their eggs, and more people are doing it each year. This expensive procedure requires collecting and storing eggs and includes taking hormone injections to stimulate egg development (see page 118) and a minimally invasive medical procedure, often under sedation. This may sound like a lot of effort for something you may never use, but it can be reassuring to know that, if you want to delay childbearing, this could be an option.

If that's you, it's worth knowing that egg freezing is not a fail-safe. There is currently only a 1-in-15 success rate for pregnancies resulting from thawed eggs. Eggs harvested before the age of 35 are statistically more viable than those collected later in life. Each country has its own rules on how long eggs can be stored or how they can be used, although there are moves to legislate for more flexibility on this.

"Navigating society's expectations is difficult. How you do—or don't—start a family is your choice."

What sort of things can affect fertility?

There are lots of reasons why people might find it difficult to conceive. In fact, issues with fertility are more common than you might expect.

Let's look at the statistics. Of 100 couples trying to conceive, 80 succeed within one year, and 10 succeed within the second year. The last 10 continue to experience fertility issues. If all those 10 couples choose to seek fertility treatment, one will remain unsuccessful.

These stats refer to people who don't expect to experience infertility. If you account for people who already know they have an issue, the proportion of people experiencing infertility is closer to one in seven.

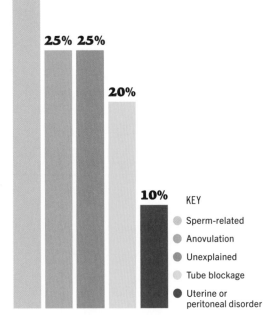

Causes of infertility

Infertility might be due to an anatomical issue. For instance, fallopian tubes can become blocked due to a build-up of scar tissue from previous surgery, pelvic inflammatory disease, or endometriosis (see page 106) in the peritoneum (body cavity). In some cases, keyhole surgery can help.

It can also be down to a lack of gametes (eggs or sperm). Anovulation (lack of ovulation) can be caused by early menopause, illness, hormonal imbalance, stress, weight, nutrition, or extreme exercise (see page 93). Many cases of infertility relate to the sperm-producing partner, but taboos sometimes prevent people from exploring this initially. And many cases remain unexplained, even after medical investigation.

Early menopause (before the age of 40) catches some people by surprise. This may be caused by illness or treatment for cancer either in childhood or adulthood (see page 143).

Other illnesses that impact fertility might be caused by hormonal irregularities. For example, hormonal conditions such as hypothyroidism or PCOS (see page 107) can disrupt ovulation.

Comparing causes of infertility

Issues with sperm, ovulation, and fallopian tubes are the most common known causes of infertility, but in many cases, the reasons remain unknown.

30% **25%** **25%** **20%** **10%**

KEY
- Sperm-related
- Anovulation
- Unexplained
- Tube blockage
- Uterine or peritoneal disorder

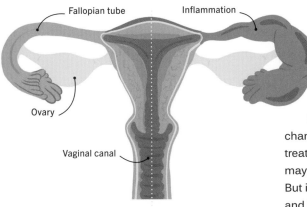

Pelvic inflammatory disease
Inflammation in the fallopian tubes and uterus can cause scar tissue to form, which blocks the path of eggs and sperm, making conception less likely.

It's worth remembering that more than one of the above factors can be present.

Improving the odds

If you're trying to conceive, the best chance you can give yourself, beyond seeking treatment for any underlying conditions you may have, is to make healthy lifestyle choices. But if you do already make sensible choices and have been trying to conceive for a while, try not to worry. Remember that, just because it takes a little longer than you might have hoped or expected, this does not mean it won't happen. In many cases, it takes a few cycles. Doctors tend not to even investigate why you haven't conceived until you've been trying for a full year.

Couples wishing to start a family can also try adoption or surrogacy. Also, fertility treatments (see pages 118–119), such as ovulation induction and IVF, may be available for those who are unable to conceive after a year of trying. For those with uterine malformations, pregnancy may still be possible, although it may take some surgical correction. Even for those who experience early menopause, donor egg IVF treatment is an option.

Hormone imbalances can also affect the thickness of the uterine lining. Trauma, both emotional and physical, as well as stress (see page 93), can delay ovulation cycles for months or even years.

Sometimes things you might not expect can affect regular cycles. Interestingly, professional athletes can find their menstrual cycles are disrupted by rigorous training schedules, and it can take a while for fertility to return to normal during and after some professional sporting careers.

If it's a sperm issue that causes infertility, it might be that the sperm count is low or that there is no sperm in semen (azoospermia). Or sperm might have poor motility, or be of poor quality due to lifestyle factors.

Healthy lifestyle choices
Do your best to eat well, keep fit and active, and avoid high stress levels while you are trying to conceive.

How do fertility treatments work?

Most people don't get to learn about fertility treatments unless they pursue them, so here's an assisted-fertility primer for those who may wish to seek help or better support a friend.

There are many reasons why people might experience infertility (see pages 116–117) and look to fertility treatments for help. Some other reasons for using fertility treatment are:

◊ **Inability to** have vaginal sex due to physical or psychosexual issues, or ejaculatory problems

◊ **Being in** a same-sex or sperm-free couple

◊ **Being single**

Thanks to technology, there are a number of fertility treatments available, with some particularly suited to specific fertility issues.

Overcoming infertility taboos

More and more people use— and discuss using—fertility treatments to become parents, so the stigma surrounding infertility is becoming a thing of the past.

Ovulation induction (OI)

OI is used in cases of anovulation and to stimulate the growth of one or more follicles (egg sacs) in the ovaries for IUI, IVF, or egg donation. Egg growth in the follicles is stimulated by either follicle-stimulating hormone (FSH) or luteinizing hormone (LH) for 10–12 days after the onset of your period. Follicle growth is then monitored by sonogram and, when it is assessed that you will soon ovulate, either you have sex, IUI is performed, or the eggs are retrieved for IVF or egg donation.

Intrauterine insemination (IUI)

IUI is used in cases of anovulation or when using donated sperm. Collected sperm is prepared in a laboratory, then deposited into the uterus via a catheter.

In vitro fertilization (IVF)

If OI combined with IUI is not successful, or in cases of low sperm count, fallopian tube blockage, or unexplained infertility, IVF is a good option. It begins with OI to stimulate the development of multiple eggs, which are then harvested from the ovaries by a small needle inserted vaginally and guided by sonogram. You may be sedated for this short (15–20-minute) procedure. The eggs are then mixed with a sufficient quantity of sperm in a petri dish in an embryology lab. Over the course of 18 hours, some of the eggs may be fertilized.

Fertilized eggs continue to develop for up to six days while the lining of the uterus is prepared for implantation by hormonal medication. One or two of the embryos are then transferred to the uterus vaginally via a catheter to enable implantation (see page 113).

Intracytoplasmic sperm injection (ICSI)

If the sperm count is low, IVF fertilization rates tend to be low as well. To improve on these rates, ICSI happens as part of the IVF process. Once the eggs are harvested, an individual sperm is physically injected into a single egg. The resulting embryo is transferred into the uterus when developmentally ready.

Using donors

In the case of a complete lack of viable eggs or sperm, donors can be used. It isn't always easy to procure these donations. The introduction of laws allowing the disclosure of the identity of the donor at the request of the adult offspring has resulted in fewer donors signing up. Both egg and sperm donors donate their gametes (eggs or sperm) altruistically to help others have a baby. Egg donors are usually fewer in number than sperm donors because the process of harvesting eggs is more invasive and impactful.

Donors are typically screened for a variety of infections and genetic diseases, and a detailed personal history is taken to ensure there is no risk of inherited disease. Sperm and egg banks exist within fertility clinics. Some people prefer to ask a friend to donate. Another source of procuring donated eggs is via egg sharing, in which a couple undergoing IVF agrees to share some of their eggs with a recipient in exchange for a reduced cost in their own treatment.

IVF using donor sperm

One cycle of IVF takes roughly three weeks to complete. Several eggs are matured and harvested. Sperm that was frozen at the point of donation is thawed before the eggs and sperm are mixed. One or two of the embryos are then transferred into the uterus, which has been primed for implantation.

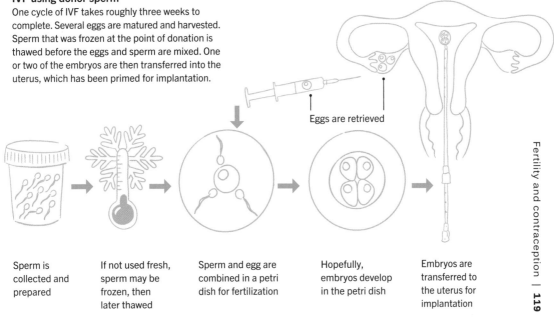

Eggs are retrieved

Sperm is collected and prepared

If not used fresh, sperm may be frozen, then later thawed

Sperm and egg are combined in a petri dish for fertilization

Hopefully, embryos develop in the petri dish

Embryos are transferred to the uterus for implantation

How do birth control pills work?

The birth control pill, which first became available in the early 1960s, is the most widely used of all prescribed forms of birth control in the US and UK.

Birth control pills are considered over 99 percent effective at preventing pregnancy *if* you use them correctly. They don't prevent STIs, so barrier methods of contraception should be used if there is a risk of infection.

There are two main types available: the combined pill and the progesterone-only pill. With either type, different brands contain various types and levels of hormones.

Combined pill

This is the most commonly prescribed type of pill. It contains estrogen and progesterone and is taken for 21 consecutive days, followed by a hormone-free interval of 7 days, during which you have a "withdrawal bleed" (see page 122). You then start the 28-day cycle again.

The combined pill delivers hormones in controlled doses each day in order to suppress ovulation. At the start of the cycle, it releases a small amount of synthetic estrogen that suppresses the release of follicle-stimulating hormone (FSH) and luteinizing hormone (LH)—the hormones that usually initiate ovulation (see pages 86–87). The progesterone that the pill contains thickens cervical mucus so sperm cannot cross the cervix. It also reduces the build-up of the lining of the uterus, making it less implantation-friendly (see page 113).

There are pros and cons to the combined pill. On the plus side, it may help reduce PMS, improve symptoms of endometriosis (see page 106), and minimize the effects of heavy and painful periods. On the minus side, certain medicines stop it from working, and there may be side effects (see pages 126–127), although some disappear once the body adjusts.

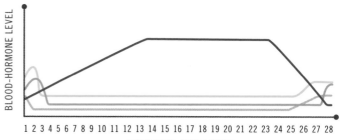

On the combined pill

This graph gives you an idea of hormone levels when on the combined pill. Estrogen levels are high after a pill-free week. The reintroduced hormones suppress the release of LH and FSH, which inhibits ovulation.

KEY — LH — Progesterone
— FSH — Estrogen

BLOOD-HORMONE LEVEL

1 2 3 4 5 6 7 8 9 10 11 12 13 14 15 16 17 18 19 20 21 22 23 24 25 26 27 28

MENSTRUAL CYCLE (DAYS)

WHEN YOU TAKE USER ERROR INTO ACCOUNT, **BIRTH CONTROL PILLS ARE 91% EFFECTIVE**

The combined pill may be unsuitable if you: are nursing; carry extra weight; smoke; have raised blood pressure; are prone to migraine or thrombosis; have disease of the liver, gall bladder, or heart; or are on any of a handful of specific medicines.

Progesterone-only pill (POP)

Also called the mini-pill, there are two types of POP. Traditional POP has one mode of action—it makes cervical mucus inhospitable to sperm. The other type (containing a type of progestogen called desogestrel) works as per traditional POP, but also suppresses ovulation. There is, however, research indicating that traditional POP also suppresses ovulation in some cases. Success rates for desogestrel POP are equal to those of the combined pill when taken correctly, while the traditional POP is slightly less effective.

The POP is taken for a full 28 days with no break. Your period will likely become irregular, infrequent, lighter, or completely stop.

This pill is suitable if you are nursing, are over the age of 35, or if you smoke. It is not for you if you have had liver disease, a stroke, or breast cancer. As with the combined pill, there may be side effects, and specific medications can reduce its efficacy.

Taking the pill

Ideally, contraceptive pills should be taken at the same time each day.

Some brands of the combined pill contain placebo pills for the hormone-free interval to help users remain in the habit of taking a pill at the same time each day. If you take the pill a full 24 hours late (so 48 hours from the last pill), this is counted as a missed pill (see page 123).

If you're over three hours late taking the traditional POP, or over 12 with the desogestrel POP, use a barrier form of contraception (see page 128) for seven days.

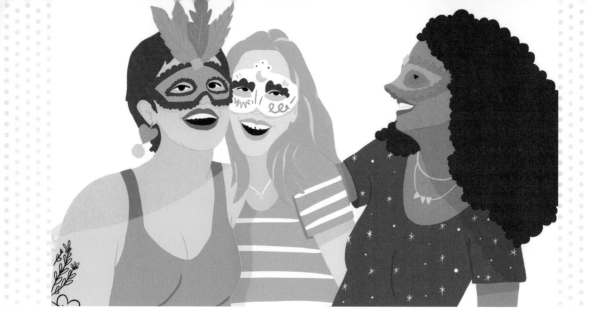

Is bleeding on the pill the same as a real period?

In a word, no. It's a totally fake period masquerading as a real one. You didn't ovulate, your uterine lining didn't build up as normal, and you're not having a real period.

Bleeding during the final week of your cycle on the combined pill is referred to as "withdrawal bleeding," caused by the withdrawal of the hormones the pill contains during the hormone-free interval (see page 120). The body sheds the lining of the uterus that has built up during that cycle. This bleed is usually shorter and lighter than a normal period due to the reduced build-up of the uterine lining when you take the pill. You may only get some light spotting, or possibly even no bleed at all.

If you want, you can skip the placebo week altogether and go straight on to the next pack—there is no clinical risk in doing this. Some people find it reassuring to have the bleed.

Some folks who are squeamish about menstrual blood may use the pill to skip periods for convenience's sake, staying on it even when they don't need contraception and aren't struggling with symptoms. Regular cycles offer a great way to monitor your health though. For tips on overcoming blood fear, see page 47.

Breakthrough bleeding

This is spotting or bleeding when you're not in the hormone-free interval and is a possible side effect of taking the pill. It should either taper off after a few months or prompt you to try another type of pill. Breakthrough bleeding should always be investigated in case it signifies cancer.

What happens if I miss a pill?

"Compliance" means taking meds as prescribed—the correct dose at the correct times—and being aware of when not to take them. It's kind of a big deal.

Not to be a party pooper, but noncompliance is a real worry when it comes to birth control, as it influences its effectiveness. (But I know there are reasons why taking your pills on schedule can be difficult—no judgment here.)

Most people on the pill use the combined pill, so the advice on this page relates to this type. Accidental noncompliance often happens by forgetting to start the next pill pack after the hormone-free interval (see page 120), and this can be an issue. Missing one pill mid-pack is not a huge problem, provided you take it as soon as you remember and take the next one on time. Bear in mind that:

◗ **The pill** can stop working after a hormone-free interval of more than eight days.
◗ **You need** to have been on the pill for seven consecutive days to be protected.

What to do

If you've missed pills, what you should do depends on how many you've missed.

If you forgot to start a new pack after the hormone-free week, and your hormone-free interval has exceeded eight days, start the new pill pack as soon as possible and use a barrier method of contraception (see page 128) until you have taken pills for seven consecutive days.

If you miss a pill mid-pack, but you've taken the pill on time for the previous seven consecutive days, take the missed pill as soon as possible. Then take the next pill at the time you would normally, even if that means taking two pills in a day, and continue with the rest of the pack as normal. No precautions are necessary.

If you've missed two or more pills, take *only* the last pill you missed as soon as possible, then take the next pill at the time you would normally and continue with the rest of the pack as usual—but use a barrier method of contraception for seven days.

If you miss two or three pills in week 3 of the pack, skip the hormone-free interval and start the next pack right after this one to ensure you have seven consecutive days of use—and use a barrier method of contraception until then.

If you were sexually active during or after the hormone-free interval and then forget to start the next pack on time or miss two to seven pills in week 1, consider emergency contraception (see page 134).

If you regularly miss pills, consider a different type of birth control (see pages 124–125).

Double up! (Occasionally)
If you miss a pill mid-pack, take it the next day, doubling up on pills for a day. The increased hormone levels may cause nausea.

Missed Friday's pill? Take it on Saturday along with Saturday's pill.

SUN   MON   TUE   WED   THU   FRI   SAT

How will the implant, ring, or patch affect me?

If you want to use hormonal birth control but the pill isn't for you, these are great low-maintenance options. They will affect your period in a similar way to the birth control pill.

As you don't have to deal with these forms of contraception daily, there's less room for error, so the hormones they deliver are more likely to do their job consistently. Because of this, they are considered to be more than 99 percent effective. Like the pill (see pages 120–121), they release estrogen and/or progesterone into the system to suppress ovulation and/or create an inhospitable environment for sperm.

As with all hormonal birth control, there may be side effects (see pages 126–127).

Three-year option
The implant is fitted beneath the skin by a medical practitioner and slowly releases hormones over a three-year period. It's not very visible, although you can see it if you look for it. Your periods generally stop entirely.

Shorter-term options
Both the contraceptive patch and the vaginal ring are replaced more frequently.

The ring is a flexible, ring-shaped device that sits high up in the vagina and releases hormones into the bloodstream continuously. You may have spotting or light bleeding at first, but this decreases over time. The patch, worn on the skin, is made of a strong, waterproof adhesive. While using the patch, your periods should become lighter and more regular.

Type of contraception	Hormone(s) released	Site of use	Frequency of replacement
Implant	Progestin (synthetic progesterone)	Inserted under the skin on the inner side of the upper arm	Replace after 3 years
Vaginal ring	Estrogen and progestin	Self-inserted into the top of the vagina	Remove after 3 weeks; follow with a ring-free week; repeat with a new ring
Contraceptive patch	Estrogen and progestin	Self-applied anywhere on the skin except on the breasts	Apply new patches weekly for 3 weeks; follow with a patch-free week; repeat

How does the IUD work, and will it affect my period?

That depends on the type of IUD you get—there are two types, and they work in slightly different ways.

Both are similarly effective T-shaped devices inserted into the uterus. Each tends to prevent implantation (see page 113).

Intrauterine device (IUD)
The IUD, or copper coil, reacts with the uterine microbiome, changing its PH and altering cervical mucus consistency. It can be left in for 5–10 years. Periods can become heavier and cramping may increase for several months.

Intrauterine system (IUS)
The IUS is made of plastic and releases progestin, which prevents pregnancy in the same way as the POP (see page 121). It can remain in place for 3–5 years. It may reduce cramps, stop periods, or make them lighter and shorter while fitted.

Risks
Each type carries a small risk of infection—see a doctor if you develop unusual discharge, a fever, or pelvic pain. There is also increased risk of ectopic pregnancy (when a fertilized egg implants in the fallopian tube instead of the uterus and must be surgically removed to prevent rupture).

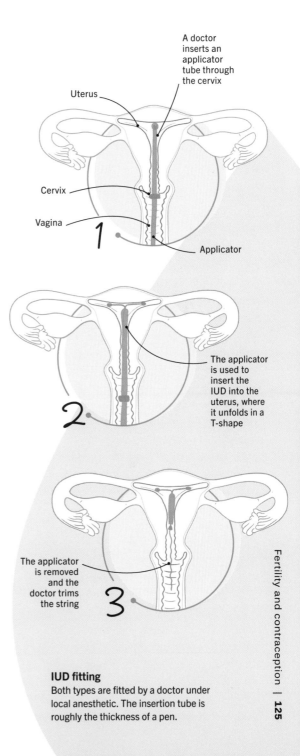

A doctor inserts an applicator tube through the cervix

Uterus

Cervix

Vagina

1

Applicator

The applicator is used to insert the IUD into the uterus, where it unfolds in a T-shape

2

The applicator is removed and the doctor trims the string

3

IUD fitting
Both types are fitted by a doctor under local anesthetic. The insertion tube is roughly the thickness of a pen.

What are the side effects of hormonal birth control?

There are several side effects linked to both taking hormonal birth control and coming off it. Changing your body's hormonal rhythms can cause physical and emotional reactions.

Hormonal contraception is incredibly helpful, whether it's the combined or progesterone-only pill (see pages 120–121), the implant, vaginal ring, or hormonal patch (see page 124), or the IUS (see page 125). Besides protecting against pregnancy, hormonal birth control can be used to treat conditions such as endometriosis, PCOS, and acne. It can also help regulate periods and heavy menstrual bleeding and provide relief from painful menstrual cramps.

But it's worth noting that there are some associated side effects. While they are not experienced by everyone, it's important to be aware of the symptoms to look out for if you are using, or are considering using, the pill or any other form of hormonal birth control. Ensure you are informed so you can make the best choices for yourself.

Noticing side effects
When you are taking hormonal contraception, it may be difficult to notice side effects at first, or you may unintentionally chalk them up to other causes. Approach your doctor for reassurance and advice if in doubt, and talk to friends or relatives about the symptoms you are experiencing.

Some doctors prescribe the same pill over and over out of habit, but each person is unique.

Ensure you find the right option for you, and don't "wait and see" for three months if you feel there's something wrong either mentally or physically. Because we are all different, hormone levels in certain hormonal birth control products may be too high for your own body's comfort.

Estrogen- and progesterone-related
Taking a large quantity of estrogen has side effects that can include: raised blood pressure, breast tenderness, headaches, nausea, indigestion, and leg cramps (ensure you rule out deep vein thrombosis). Don't take birth control containing estrogen if you or your family has a history of blood clots or if you develop high blood pressure.

Finding your equilibrium
It might take a little trial and error to find the right product for you. Be alert to side effects. And be confident—don't be afraid to ask your doctor to help you find a better fit.

Taking a large quantity of progesterone has side effects that can include: mood swings, depression, breast tenderness, swelling, acne, nausea, and vomiting.

Coming off

When you come off hormonal birth control, you may find your cervical mucus changes as your body releases excess estrogen.

There have been some interesting studies looking at the effects of pill-controlled cycles. One study found that some pill-takers were less sexually attracted to their partners once they came off the pill.

Another study showed that, on natural cycles, women who were attracted to men reported finding them more attractive if they had softer features and baby faces for most of the cycle, but were interested in more rugged-looking ones around the fertile window (see page 113). It was posited in the journal article that, during ovulation, they were attracted to people with features of higher levels of testosterone—meaning it's possible that the sorts of people you find attractive might change when you start supressing ovulation.

Both studies suggest that hormonal birth control alters feelings that we might experience in a natural cycle.

What are some nonchemical forms of birth control?

If you've had bad experiences with hormonal contraception, or if you've decided it simply isn't for you, there are other options.

Unless you're interested in trying something like the Fertility Awareness Method (see opposite), there are two main routes for you if you're looking for birth control options that don't involve taking hormones.

Sterilization

Permanent or near-permanent birth-control procedures are preferred by those who intend to be child-free or who have children but don't plan to have more. These procedures do not affect hormonal or sexual function. They include:

◊ **Tubal ligation**—surgery to block off the fallopian tubes from the uterus so that eggs cannot be fertilized.

◊ **Vasectomy**—surgery to block off the testes so that semen no longer contains sperm.

Barrier methods

These place a physical barrier between egg and sperm to prevent fertilization, and they can be highly effective if used correctly. Condoms are a popular choice, as they also offer protection against most STIs.

Even if you're using hormonal birth control or have had a permanent procedure, if you have casual partners of any gender, you're at risk of catching or passing on STIs. So it's important to also use a barrier method of contraception when engaging in oral, anal, or genital contact or when sharing sex toys. Barriers include:

◊ **External condoms**—the familiar sort of condom worn on the penis or placed on a penetrative sex toy.

◊ **Internal condoms**—a less common design worn inside the vagina or placed inside a penetrable sex toy.

PREVENTING STIs

There are a number of measures you can take to avoid STIs:

◊ **Use barrier forms** of contraception during higher-risk sexual activities such as genital, anal, and oral contact.

◊ **Always wash sex toys** before use and when sharing between partners.

◊ **Before having** sex with a new partner, discuss herpes status (it's a common infection), compare notes on when you were last tested for other STIs, and disclose any positive infection status.

◊ **Get tested** regularly for STIs. Seek treatment early if diagnosed.

Can I use cycle-charting as contraception or to become pregnant?

You can—to a point. The Fertility Awareness Method (FAM) is used as a way of preventing or timing pregnancy, but it's more effective for the latter.

FAM is a holistic method for tracking the subtle changes in your body to predict when you're most fertile (see page 112), so that you can choose your sexual activity to match, depending on whether you want to conceive or prevent pregnancy.

One factor FAM picks up on is the surge in luteinizing hormone (see pages 86–87) that stimulates your ovaries to produce an egg. However, there's no guarantee you'll be able to determine when you've ovulated using this technique. Because bodies aren't 100 percent predictable and our observation skills aren't 100 percent accurate, FAM does have its limits, particularly when it comes to preventing pregnancy. Many people also use home ovulation testing kits and smart thermometers to track their fertility and conceive.

Finding resources and support

There are a number of organizations and training programs that teach people how to use these methods or that offer the support of a professional. Justisse is one of the international networks of holistic reproductive health practitioners (HRHPs) looking to reclaim reproductive healthcare from highly medicalized practices that can seem inaccessible or depersonalizing.

FAM practitioners work in many countries around the world, including the US, teaching the methods of observing natural cycles to their clients. Having a guide can be very reassuring, if you want to try this approach.

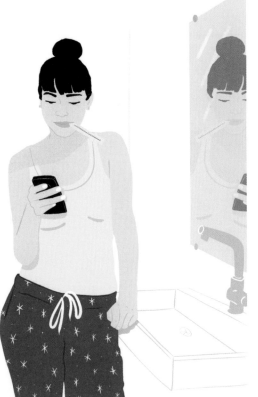

Can you get pregnant during your period?

Potentially, yes, so it's best to track your cycle (see pages 90–91) and look out for the signs of ovulation. Bodies can have a mind of their own ...

You might be regularly ovulating earlier or later in your cycle than you think you are—the luteal phase (see page 89) isn't exactly 14 days long. That's just an estimate.

It's not that common, but you can also ovulate twice during a cycle. Usually, your ovaries are predictable, with one releasing a single egg at around the midpoint of your cycle.

They usually play fair and do this only once per cycle, but sometimes one goes rogue and starts growing another egg follicle, and we don't know why. So if you are having sex during your period with someone who produces sperm or did so during the week before the rogue ovulation—boom!

If you'd rather not take the risk, use a barrier method of contraception or consider other types of play during your period, or look into long-term birth control options like the pill (see page 120).

Remember that withdrawal isn't a surefire way of preventing pregnancy, as preejaculate can contain viable sperm.

Track your cycle

It's a good idea to monitor your cycle (see pages 90–91), whether you're trying to get pregnant or not. It's a great way to get comfortable with recognizing your regular pattern of fertile signs (see page 112), as well as premenstrual signs. And it can keep you aware of your body and help you feel more liberated in the bedroom.

Can you be pregnant and still have a period?

No, not an actual menstrual period—but you can experience light bleeding or spotting, which you might confuse for a period, especially if it happens regularly.

On occasion, people continue to have what *appear* to be periods throughout a pregnancy, only to find out later in the pregnancy that these were not periods after all. In such cases, it may be abnormal bleeding in pregnancy, and it's unlikely that the bleeds are exactly cyclical, but they might happen regularly enough to seem like a menstrual cycle.

The reasons for bleeding in very early pregnancy are unknown, but it's thought there is a rupture of blood vessels during the implantation of a fertilized egg (see page 113), as the embryo embeds itself into lining of the uterus, that may cause spotting.

Late discovery

Although the media tends to sensationalize unexpected births and focus on the few cases where it only becomes obvious during the labor and delivery, such cases are rare. However, discovering your pregnancy once you're already partway through it isn't so uncommon.

Being unaware of a pregnancy is less than ideal for a number of reasons. It can mean termination is no longer possible. Even if you are happy to be pregnant, your less-than-pregnancy-aware lifestyle may have impacted the early development of a fetus if it included alcohol or recreational drugs. And you may have missed opportunities to take prenatal vitamins and screen for or treat health issues in both you and the fetus.

Discovering a pregnancy in its later stages is related to a higher risk of adverse outcomes, so if there is a chance you could become pregnant, stay tuned into your body and your cycle, keeping an eye out for the signs of pregnancy (see page 132).

Staying pregnant

There are a few precautions you can take if you get, and intend to stay, pregnant. Avoid spending too long in hot tubs and saunas, which can be risky. Also avoid alcohol, cigarettes, nicotine, and nonprescribed drugs. Ensure you eat a healthy diet, and include folic acid supplements, as this has been proven to support fetal brain and spinal development.

Don't ignore heavy bleeding

Light bleeding in early pregnancy is not uncommon, but if you experience heavy bleeding at any stage, consult a doctor immediately, as it might be a sign of a complication.

What are some early signs I might be pregnant?

There are lots of signs of pregnancy to look out for, but some people don't experience any symptoms at all, and others mistake them for PMS. If in doubt, pick up a pregnancy test.

If you chart your cycle regularly, it will help you identify when you might have ovulated, which will help you work out what the approximate date of conception was if you're pregnant. Without that valuable piece of data, how many weeks pregnant you are is calculated from the first day of your last period. This means that, weirdly, you'd be considered four weeks pregnant before you even start noticing any signs of pregnancy, such as a missed period.

In fact, let's start there. Signs you might detect from conception to two weeks later are:

◊ **A missing** period. About that: if you didn't intend to become pregnant but realized mid-cycle that you had unprotected sex within your fertile window (see page 113), the panic of that discovery alone may have delayed ovulation. A missed period might not be a pregnancy, but instead a late period, because you threw off your cycle's timings with your stress. However, for many people, a missed period is the main sign to look out for, and it is still the big indicator.

◊ **A much** lighter period or just spotting. You may notice spotting and wonder if that is your period, but it could be implantation bleeding—a couple of spots of pink or red blood that can appear when the egg implants in the wall of the uterus. This happens close to when your period would be due.

◊ **Mood swings** or feeling extra sensitive or anxious. Could it be PMS? Or a surge of pregnancy hormones? Who knows?!

◊ **A positive** pregnancy test. It's very easy to get a negative test if you've not had much build-up of pregnancy hormones yet. Some "early" tests that guarantee to provide accurate results may not live up to their promises, so you should definitely test again about a week after an early negative test if you still haven't had your period. There are rarely false positives.

Other indicators that you may start to notice during the first three months of the pregnancy include:

◊ **Being affected** by strong food smells

◊ **Feeling bloated** or queasy regularly, particularly in the mornings

◊ **Painful or** tender breasts

◊ **Needing to** pee more than usual

◊ **Feeling *really*** tired

Period or pregnant?

Early signs are identical to how you feel when your period is due, which can be either frustrating or terrifying, depending on if you do or don't want the pregnancy.

"Whether you are pregnant or not, remember that you need love, care, and nurturing, so treat yourself well."

How does emergency contraception work?

There are some myths surrounding emergency contraception, so let's bust those first. You don't have to go to the ER to get it, or rush out to get it as soon as you've had sex!

Depending on the type you choose, emergency contraception should be taken within up to five days of unprotected sex. There are no issues with taking it more than once in your life. In fact, you may need to if you rely on barrier methods of birth control, as these can sometimes fail. But if you find yourself relying on it, consider another form of contraception (see pages 120–125). You may find that it saves you time and money and is much easier on your hormones.

Pill form

Two types of emergency contraception come in pill form. One works best if taken within three days of sexual contact, and the other within five days. Both work by preventing ovulation.

The five-day pill is slightly more effective but is prescription only. Usually, there are few side effects, but if you vomit soon after taking either pill, you may need to take it again.

IUD

The IUD can also be requested at your doctor's office or a sexual health clinic as emergency contraception. This prevents implantation of a fertilized egg (see page 113). It should be inserted by a doctor within five days of sexual contact. The IUD may cause cramps or bleeding and, in rare cases, infection, just as it would if you were not using it in an emergency (see page 125). It has an added benefit—it can remain in the uterus as ongoing contraception.

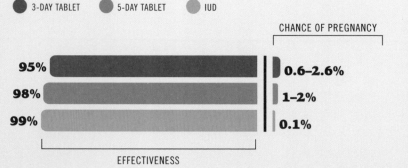

● 3-DAY TABLET   ● 5-DAY TABLET   ● IUD

CHANCE OF PREGNANCY

95%   0.6–2.6%

98%   1–2%

99%   0.1%

EFFECTIVENESS

Effectiveness
The IUD is the most effective form of emergency contraception, followed by the 5-day tablet, then the 3-day tablet— but all three are generally reliable.

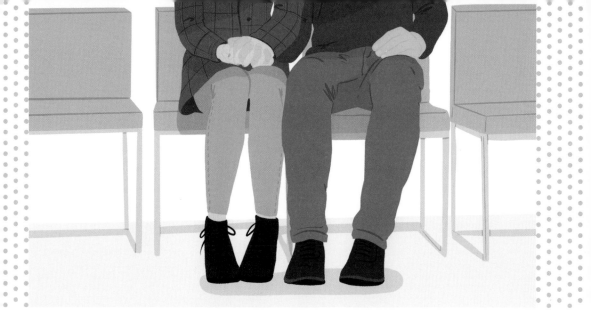

What if I choose to end a pregnancy?

Termination is an emotional and stigmatized issue, which is challenging to navigate if it is what you choose. Put your well-being first and make your decision based on your needs.

Some people who choose termination feel pragmatic about it, while others are conflicted. Either way, it helps to reach out for support from a friend or reputable nonprofit organization.

There are two types of termination: medical and surgical. Medical termination can take place from conception to the point at which the fetus is considered "viable," which varies from country to country. During this type of termination, you are given two drugs to take 48 hours apart—the first orally, the second either orally or vaginally. You are given painkillers and can expect bleeding and a lot of cramping, both of which settle in 7–10 days. See a doctor if these side effects don't go away, as this may be a sign of tissue remaining in the uterus or of infection.

Surgical termination can take place from conception to 12 weeks. Anesthetic is administered for this procedure. The cervix is dilated and a cannula is inserted to remove the fetus. After a surgical termination, it is also normal to bleed for about 7–10 days. If done in an appropriately sterile hospital environment, the procedure is reasonably safe, but it should be noted that anytime the cervix is dilated and instruments are introduced, there is a risk of infection. There is also a small risk of uterine perforation.

How can I tell an early miscarriage from a late period?

If a miscarriage takes place around the time you would have had your period, it's hard to tell the difference unless you happen to have taken a pregnancy test.

An early miscarriage that takes place right after implantation (see page 113) is called a chemical pregnancy, because pregnancy hormones may show up on a test—but there is no viable pregnancy. Signs of early miscarriage are cramping and spotting (or what looks like a period, possibly with more clots than usual).

If you were not planning to become pregnant, you may be totally unaware of the miscarriage. However, uncertainty about whether or not you've miscarried, or despair over a lost pregnancy (if you've already taken a test), can be overwhelming. It is absolutely no consolation, of course, but it is worth knowing that a pregnancy ending so soon was most likely not one that would have continued to term for a number of reasons, such as hormonal or genetic problems. Early miscarriages that happen for this reason generally cannot be prevented.

Causes of later miscarriages are varied, and some remain unexplained. Seek medical help if you experience heavy bleeding, cramping, pain, or nausea.

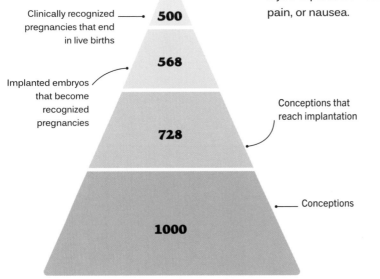

Clinically recognized pregnancies that end in live births — **500**

568

Implanted embryos that become recognized pregnancies

Conceptions that reach implantation

728

Conceptions

1000

Rate of miscarriage
Many fertilized eggs will not make it to implantation. They are lost before a pregnancy is even discovered and mistaken for a late period. Research indicates that only half of all fertilized eggs actually result in live births.

How common are stillbirth and late miscarriage?

More common than you might think. But you may never hear about them, because of the taboos around reproductive health combined with those surrounding death and bereavement.

You may have friends and relatives who have experienced miscarriage or stillbirth, and who never speak of their experiences. For generations, taboos were upheld that defined the loss of a baby as being a "failure" of some kind. Tragically, in the past, miscarried or stillborn babies were considered "not real people," and parents were often encouraged to move on from the experience immediately. All too often, deceased babies were swiftly removed by labor ward attendants.

More recently, advocacy groups and research into social and cultural attitudes to late miscarriage and stillbirth have begun to create new ways of responding to such events. Outdated attitudes are starting to change.

Now, in hospitals, protocols include supporting parents to spend time with their stillborn baby, name them, dress them, take handprints and footprints as keepsakes, and take photos of them and with them – all to ensure there are many touchstones for talking and sharing memories in the future. Many hospitals have designed bereavement suites with the help of patients, researchers, and staff on the wards to ensure that families have a private space to grieve and to acknowledge and celebrate a difficult but nonetheless unique and important birth experience.

Some families go on to have more children, known, delightfully, as "rainbow babies," as they are considered to have arrived like the rainbow after the storm.

For the past few years, many celebrities have shared openly their grief and joy at becoming proud parents to babies who have sadly died. Such public examples help open up the conversation for everyone.

1 IN 160

BIRTHS IN THE US IS A **STILLBIRTH**. THE MAJORITY ARE **UNEXPLAINED**.

Whether you are talking to someone who has experienced stillbirth or late miscarriage or have gone through one yourself, don't be afraid to ask questions or mention a baby who has passed away. Don't presume that this person or experience is or should be a secret.

The fact is, though, that much more research is needed into the causes of late miscarriage and stillbirth. If this issue has affected you, a family member, or a friend, there are many support and advocacy organizations you or they can reach out to, even if the loss happened many years ago.

Is the bleed right after having a baby a period?

No, it's called postpartum bleeding. It can take some people by surprise, as it doesn't get talked about much, but it's good to know about it in advance, as it's a full-on bloody experience!

Right after giving birth, the body sheds the uterine lining and a bunch of mucus in an epic bleed. The stuff the uterus expels is referred to as lochia, and there's so much of it that many people use reusable or disposable postpartum pads or period underwear that are as thick as nighttime menstrual pads.

Postpartum bleeding often continues for 3–10 days, followed by 4–6 weeks of lighter bleeding, then spotting, then discharge.

Many people don't know about lochia until they have a baby themselves. The combination of menstrual taboos, pregnancy taboos, and the rose-tinted view caused by birth hormones leads many new parents to just not mention it.

If you're planning to have a baby, lochia is something you should know about, not just because it's interesting, but also because it can be scary if you're not expecting it. And you can't prepare for what you don't know about, especially at a time when you'll have lots of other things on your mind. Some people find they don't menstruate for a while if they're nursing, but they will experience this potentially unexpected bleeding, even if they gave birth by C-section. So be mentally and physically prepared. And spread the word!

At the ready

To be ready for postpartum bleeding, have cloth pads, period underwear, or disposable pads handy. You may want to have or make a set of seat pads for the first week or so—you never know how long you'll be in one spot with a milk-drunk baby passed out on your shoulder, limiting your opportunities to get up to change pads. New routines, depleted energy, and mobility issues if you've had a C-section or other complications may also limit you. Don't use tampons, as you're at a heightened risk of infection while your cervix is still partially open as it returns to roughly its normal size and shape.

Do periods change once you've had a baby?

They may be different after pregnancy. This is part of a natural change as you age and is also affected by how hormones resettle after pregnancy, as well as physical changes.

Unless you are exclusively nursing, your cycle is likely to fall back into a regular rhythm a couple of months after childbirth. If you had a perineal tear or anal fissure during childbirth, stay alert in your first few cycles for extra pain, bleeding, or a burning sensation, as these could be signs of further injury or infection. Hopefully all will be well, although, as the cycles roll by, you may notice a few differences.

Flow or length

Once your cycle settles down, you might find that your periods have become heavier, last longer, or feel painful. This may be because the uterus, having become larger for a time (it shrinks back to nearly its prepregnancy size in about 6 weeks), develops a larger endometrial lining each cycle to shed.

Cramps may become less painful. This may be due to the cervix and uterus having become more stretched and relaxed by pregnancy.

Cycles do gradually shorten and lighten over time as we age, but they can get heavier again during perimenopause (see page 142).

Bleeding angle

If you use external menstrual products, you might find that your menstrual blood no longer hits the product in the same position as it did prior to pregnancy, especially if you had a vaginal birth. The way your pelvic floor now

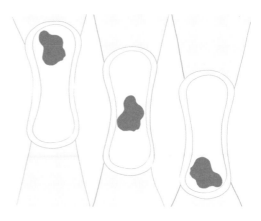

How do you bleed?
Are you a front, middle, or back bleeder? Position your menstrual pad in the gusset of your underwear accordingly.

sits, or the way your vaginal opening rests in your vulva, may mean that the route your blood or discharge takes out of the vagina is slightly altered (see above). You might find that you were a front bleeder who is now a middle bleeder, or that you were a middle bleeder who has become a back bleeder.

When discovering this change, some have the fear that their vagina or vulva is forever changed. But it's not—you'll still recognize your vulva if you look in a mirror. You've just found a new groove, is all, and all you need to do is alter the positioning of your external menstrual product.

Perimenopause and menopause

Just as menstruation has a fascinating origin story, it also has a thrillingly climactic ending. Don't believe all the negative hype around the end of periods—this chapter debunks myths and deconstructs the science on a part of life that we as a society should really understand a lot better. Learn how we can harness new knowledge about menopause to create an empowered future.

How will my period change throughout my life?

The menovulatory span (see page 114) is unique to each menstruator, but there are a few key steps along the way that most people will recognize.

When you start menstruating, at first cycles are irregular but will even out. Into your twenties, you have regular cycles and hit peak fertility. Your cycles remain the same into your thirties. In your mid-thirties, fertility begins to wane, but your cycles remain regular. In your forties, cycles may become shorter and your period may become heavier when you reach perimenopause (which is the stage leading up to menopause and the end of the menovulatory span).

Menopause transition

Perimenopause can begin at different ages and varies in length. You are still fertile during perimenopause, as your ovaries still produce eggs, but reserves are low, and reproductive hormones wind down. Skipped cycles slowly increase in frequency until, eventually, periods cease. Menopausal symptoms (see page 146) may occur in late perimenopause.

Menopause itself is not a stage, but a moment—when you have your last period. You can only know it in hindsight—a year after your last period if you were over 50 when you had it, or two years, if you were under 50. You may still experience symptoms of hormonal fluctuations, but you no longer ovulate or menstruate and you are therefore considered postmenopausal.

Menstrual cycles from start to finish
Starting out irregular, cycles settle into a regular pattern until perimenopause, after which they become variable again until they stop completely.

Pre-puberty	Reproductive years			Perimenopause			Post-menopause
	EARLY	PEAK	LATE	EARLY	LATE		
	Variable to regular	Regular	Regular	Variable 🔴 Cycles become shorter	Variable 🔴 Skipped cycles 🔴 Periods become heavier	1 year without a period	

First menstrual period (menarche)

Last menstrual period (menopause)

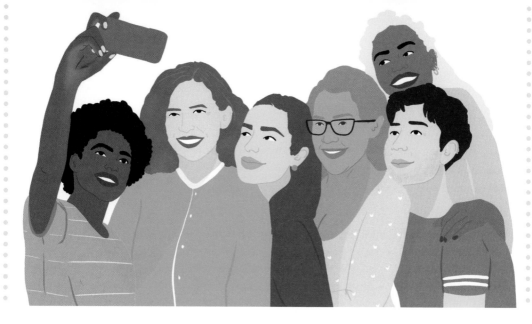

What are some other reasons why periods might stop permanently?

There are a number of medical conditions that can result in menopause arriving sooner than expected. Menopause before the age of 40 is known as premature ovarian insufficiency.

Let's start with something positive: childhood cancer survival rates have risen to 80 percent in North America, the UK, and western Europe. This is a huge advantage of successful treatments that cure a number of childhood cancers. The unintended negative, though, is that many of these treatments can affect fertility later in life and can put people into early menopause.

Gender transition

Masculinizing hormone therapy gradually ends periods.

Rare situations

Turner syndrome (a chromosomal condition) may cause accelerated egg follicle breakdown and is often associated with early menopause. Menopause may also be triggered by a hysterectomy or an oophorectomy (removal of the uterus and ovaries). For example, surgery for womb-related cancers can result in menopause, as can surgical treatments for gender reassignment, endometriosis, or fibroids. In rare cases, an autoimmune condition can instigate the onset of menopause.

Why do people view menopause negatively?

Just like periods, menopause has been shrouded in mystery and fear for centuries. It's yet another taboo subject that needs serious reclaiming!

The myths about this ordinary life stage abound, so let's break some of them down.

Symptoms aren't always awful

First of all, not everyone has a terrible menopause. Some people barely notice the transition. Symptoms (see page 146) don't go on forever. Once you stop ovulating for good, hormones settle down again, and you're back on an even keel.

You're not somehow diminished

Some people are sad to see their periods go, while others are relieved not to have to deal with them again. Either way, the end of menstruating and your fertile years doesn't make you, somehow, less of a person. You are not your fertility, and your menstrual cycle does not define your gender identity or expression. And that means anyone can celebrate or bemoan their own period—or its demise—whatever their age or gender.

You're not suddenly "old"

Statistically, about half the people born today will live to 100—which means they could spend half their life postmenopausal. As we are redefining aging as a culture right now, it's best to leave behind the myth that being menopausal means you're old—or that old is bad. That idea is so last century.

DEFY MIXED MESSAGES

Isn't it funny how society is so focused on people who don't menstruate, then ignores postmenopausal people? No. It's not.

For decades of their lives, menstruators are encouraged to pretend they don't menstruate. When they finally stop, they find themselves in a society that makes older people feel invisible and worthless.

One factor that's responsible for this is that menstrual-product manufacturers have much less to sell to someone who doesn't menstruate. So their value as a consumer becomes nonexistent—and so do they! Suddenly, postmenopausal folk become another marginalized group.

Remember that menstruating you is no better than menopausal you. Ignore the fact that society focuses like heck on the middle part of life and think about yours holistically. Experience each stage of your life for what it truly is—as defined by you.

That's not it for sex

Your sex life doesn't end with the last of your eggs. It may be reported that there is some loss of libido, but there are some excellent workarounds for those who seek them, and many people don't need them. Some enjoy sex more once there's no risk of pregnancy.

How should we talk about menopause?

Openly. Actively break the taboos that keep this subject an unspoken reality. If you're menopausal, talk about it. If you're not, ask about it.

We need to talk about menopause more. We need to see more menopausal people on TV and in movies. In fact, we need to become more literate about aging in general, and the signs that we are reaching different milestones through life's equally glorious stages.

We need to make workplaces menopause-friendly and learn how to talk about perimenopause with our friends and families *way* before it starts—just as we are learning to do with periods. The menovulatory span of life (see page 114) isn't our entire life.

More research and education is needed on the causes of the physical aspects of perimenopause. The more accurately and openly we talk about this, the more we will be creating a culture in which we can organize and influence attitudes and policy—in medicine, in the workplace, in government ... everywhere.

Influencing the symptoms

Yes, we've all heard about how rough the symptoms of perimenopause and menopause can be (see page 146). But believe it or not, the worse you feel about menopause, the worse your menopause symptoms feel. For real! There have been studies of people experiencing perimenopausal symptoms, in which those who reported negative attitudes to menopause or aging, and worried about managing the symptoms they anticipated, reported worse symptoms than those who did not fear aging or managing menopause.

According to a survey by the British Menopause Society in 2016, only 50 percent of people surveyed who had perimenopausal symptoms discussed them with a doctor. It doesn't have to be this way.

What are the changes I might experience during perimenopause and how can I manage them?

There are a bunch of symptoms you might experience as hormones fluctuate before and during menopause, and most can be addressed. So what can you expect?

The drop in estrogen levels that occurs perimenopausally impacts the hypothalamus, causing physical and emotional side effects. Most people get a few symptoms, others get lots, and some seem to have none at all. But for the majority, there'll be obvious changes:

◊ **Shorter periods**, then shorter cycles. Periods may be lighter and preceded by a day or two of spotting. Eventually, they tend to get heavier, and some people describe "flooding"—an extremely heavy period arriving like a crimson wave.

◊ **Night sweats** and hot flashes. These are sudden rushes of higher internal temperature caused by the hypothalamus regulating your temperature inconsistently.

◊ **Insomnia due** to temperature changes (see above) and also due to changes to your circadian rhythm (the internal mechanism that regulates your sleep–wake cycle).

◊ **Dry skin** and vaginal dryness, potentially leading to painful sex.

◊ **Low sex** drive due to a combination of vaginal dryness, lack of sleep, and lower testosterone levels (see page 151).

◊ **Acne and** rosacea can increase, and you can develop changes in skin pigmentation—lighter skin tones in particular show dark spots.

◊ **More urgency** to pee and decreased muscle tone in your pelvic floor, which can lead to minor incontinence or prolapse if not addressed.

◊ **Weight gain** around your core and in your breasts.

◊ **A change** in the texture of your hair and loss of its pigmentation (and this can happen anywhere on your body).

◊ **Joint aches**, plus a decrease in bone density, potentially leading to pain and fractures.

◊ **Forgetfulness and** a lack of focus.

◊ **Mood changes**, as in PMS (see page 98). Internalized stigma; pressure at work to manage menopause in silence; and, if you're unlucky, a less-than-supportive partner

Catalysts

Symptoms can often influence and amplify one another—for instance, not sleeping properly can make you feel more irritable.

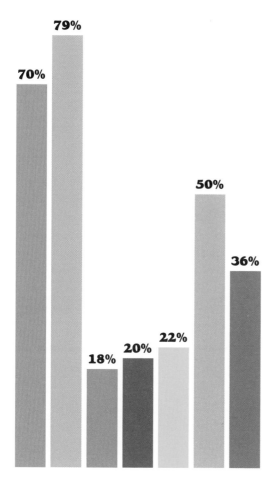

79%

70%

50%

36%

22%

18% **20%**

KEY

● Night sweats

● Hot flashes

● Achy joints

● Issues with memory or concentration

○ Insomnia

● Sex life impacted

● Social life impacted

Prevalence of symptoms
The above percentages, collected by the British Menopause Society in 2016, represent how many of those surveyed reported each symptom.

can all magnify difficult symptoms, with potential consequences for your well-being and relationships.

Adjusting to changes

So what can you do? Start a few good habits now. You can aim to prevent outcomes like incontinence and prolapse by doing regular pelvic floor exercises (see page 76) and strengthening your core. Charting your cycle (see pages 90–91) is a good idea, as is adopting a daily skincare routine, healthy diet, and regular bedtime. An honest, communicative relationship and a manageable workload will help, too.

These things can all be continued once symptoms begin. You could also consider aesthetic changes that make you feel good, such as a new hair color or tidy facial hair management. A lot of perimenopausal folks dress in lots of thin layers and carry a hand fan, stripping down, cardiganning up, and fanning at will when hot flashes happen. And invest in plenty of moisturizer and lube to alleviate dryness both outside and in. You can also ask your doctor about a hormonal prescription to manage symptoms (see page 148), and many people do.

There are things you can do beyond the personal, too., such as getting your workplace set up with a menopause policy. This could allow employees to manage temperatures where they are stationed; keep a bottle of water with them; support the sleep patterns of shift workers; and offer breaks, flextime, or adaptable uniforms. It's important to not presume that all jobs and industries are the same when it comes to managing perimenopause at work.

What is HRT? Is it safe?

Hormone replacement therapy (HRT) has been shown to be an effective form of treatment for perimenopausal symptoms, but the practice can still seem a little mysterious.

HRT involves replacing estrogen in the recipient's body as they produce less during menopause. Fluctuating estrogen levels are responsible for most common perimenopausal symptoms (see pages 146–147), including hot flashes, mood swings, and achy joints. HRT provides a steady amount of estrogen, so overall levels fall more gradually, reducing symptoms.

Along with estrogen, people undergoing HRT are prescribed progestins to stop the uterine lining from continuing to grow. This can help prevent womb-related cancers and reduce flooding (see page 146).

Taking HRT

There are several sorts of HRT, containing different amounts and types of estrogen and progestin, and it can take time to find the one that suits you best. HRT can be taken orally in the form of tablets or transdermally via a patch or a gel, often applied on the thighs.

As with the contraceptive pill (see pages 120–121), it takes a few months for your body to settle into any type of HRT. There's no upper limit for how long you can stay on it, though it's not recommended to begin HRT for the first time after the age of 60, because the risks (which we'll get to in a bit) increase with age.

HRT can be either "continuous combined" or "sequential." In the former, you take both estrogen and progestin daily. This is best for people who haven't had a period for a year or two (in other words, postmenopausal folks), because it can cause breakthrough bleeding if you're still producing estrogen. In sequential

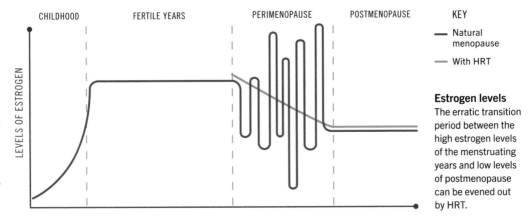

LEVELS OF ESTROGEN

CHILDHOOD   FERTILE YEARS   PERIMENOPAUSE   POSTMENOPAUSE

KEY

— Natural menopause

— With HRT

Estrogen levels
The erratic transition period between the high estrogen levels of the menstruating years and low levels of postmenopause can be evened out by HRT.

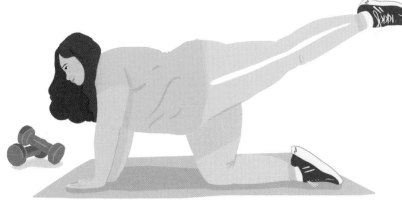

Staying active
HRT has been shown to help keep bones strong, allowing people to maintain active lives after menopause.

HRT, you take estrogen daily and progestin for 12–14 days per month. It's advised for those who are perimenopausal, and causes regular withdrawal bleeds (see page 122).

If you have queries or want more detailed care, seek out a reputable menopause specialist.

Pros and cons

There are many proven benefits of HRT. As well as controlling perimenopausal symptoms, it helps prevent osteoporotic fractures and may even protect against heart disease and bowel cancer. Because of these benefits, HRT is especially recommended for those undergoing premature menopause (menopause before the age of 40).

The side effects, however, have sometimes been misreported. In the past, there has been panic over potential risks of breast cancer, stroke, and blood clots, which encouraged many people to stop taking or prescribing HRT or to try less effective and less regulated remedies. More recent research suggests that the day-to-day risks and losses associated with perimenopause symptoms are higher than the slightly elevated risks of these other conditions.

These days, there are menopause and public health messaging organizations that stay on top of best practice, new research, and accurate reporting to help us make informed choices, such as the Society for Menstrual Cycle Research. Recent studies show that there is a real improvement in the quality of life reported by patients taking HRT within the first few years of the onset of perimenopause.

Oh, and be aware of the potentially misleading use of the phrases "compounded HRT" and "bioidentical HRT." Some are marketed as health supplements rather than medicines, so they may not have undergone the scrutiny and safety tests of a regulatory agency such as the FDA in the US.

Can I still get pregnant if I'm menopausal?

As surprising as it might sound, it is possible to get pregnant even when you're menopausal—it just means you're not postmenopausal.

Technically, menopause is defined as the time when the menstrual cycle has stopped. The thing is, though, it's not defined at the time, but in retrospect. You may think you've finished going through perimenopause, but if you still have some eggs and some hormones, then pregnancy is still possible, despite erratic or absent bleeds. Lots of folks have had (or have been) a surprise pregnancy during perimenopause—a "change-of-life baby," as it used to be called.

A pregnancy later in life can be incredibly uplifting for those who were hoping to conceive at this stage but crushing for someone who never wished to be pregnant or had decided to stop having children. Ending the pregnancy may be difficult to navigate, with other generations potentially wanting to be involved in the process. Continuing the pregnancy can mean rethinking finances or life plans. It can also be a health risk for those with additional comorbidities or chronic conditions due to age, genetics, or lifestyle. On a happier note, though, both cultural attitudes and medical advances around maternal age are improving as lifespans increase.

CONCEIVING NATURALLY DURING THE MENOPAUSAL TRANSITION
IS RARE
BUT STILL POSSIBLE

Remain alert

Some of the early symptoms of pregnancy, such as mood swings and absent periods, can be easily confused for signs of perimenopause. It's a good idea to go on charting your cycle during perimenopause to keep track of symptoms like these (see page 132).

Continue using contraception if you already do (and of course, keep using condoms to protect from STIs, if needed). How long you continue to ovulate in later life is different for everyone, but doctors generally advise to keep using contraception for at least one year after your last period if you're over 50, and two years if you're under 50.

In touch with your body

Stay tuned into the cues your body gives you, even when you think you've moved beyond the risk of pregnancy.

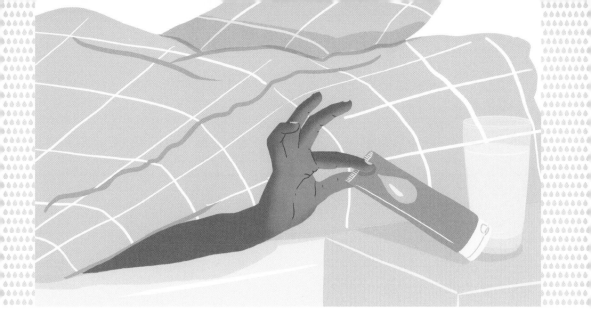

Does sex feel different after my periods stop?

Changes to sex drive and vaginal lubrication are common side effects of menopause. But feeling "different" doesn't have to mean feeling "bad."

Both changing hormone levels and the pressure of dealing with perimenopause can reduce libido. This issue can be multifaceted and shouldn't be dismissed as unfixable or your "fault." Many menopausal people experience vaginal dryness due to reduced estrogen levels. You can be prescribed vaginal estrogen to address this. There are also nonhormonal vaginal moisturizers that can be applied regularly. To supplement reduced levels of arousal fluid during sex, use plenty of extra lube!

Getting your groove back

If you're in a relationship with a non-menstruator or someone premenopausal,

have a heart-to-heart about what you're dealing with. Relearn what feels good—your vaginal landscape is changing, which means you get to explore it all over again.

If low libido is impacting your well-being, speak to your doctor. If the cause is hormonal, the British Menopause Society recommends starting with HRT (see pages 148–149) and adding testosterone, which is so far unlicensed in the UK and the US, but may be used under the supervision of a doctor. If you think the cause of your low sex drive is nonhormonal, it's worth asking to be referred to a sex therapist.

"The next chapter is up to you."

What comes after menopause?

The rest of your magnificent life, that's what! The future is not the doom and gloom that menopause taboos would have you believe.

I'm serious. There are now a growing number of studies, reports, and first-hand accounts from experts who research menopause and have presented and logged lots of qualitative data to back this up. Life after periods can be pretty great.

The next life stage

Chemically, when you reach this stage of life, your body has changed: the hormones you had before were geared toward a purpose you probably no longer need (getting pregnant). Many postmenopausal folks report an amazing sense of freedom.

This isn't to say that postmenopausal you is better or even different from menstruating you. The truth is that you're equally important whether or not you're regularly bleeding.

Societal attitudes

Despite huge strides forward over the last century, our society is still pretty uneven—in lots of ways. Most of the people who have babies also do the bulk of the emotional labor required to look after them; in many parts of the world, policy dictates that fetuses are more important than the people who carry them; and the belief persists that work done outside the home is more important than that done inside it.

A lot of people say that, after menopause, the desire to engage with the cultural pressure to primarily be a nurturer and people-pleaser fades hard, even for those people who happily dote on children or get really into community work. There's a weight off their shoulders, and I'm reliably told that it can feel fantastic!

As awesome as they are, your menstrual cycles are not you. Your whole *life* is a cycle, and embracing that is the real power as you enjoy whatever comes next.

Social pressure

The mixed messages that we receive as menstruators can be complicated to navigate and hard to reconcile with our personal choices and even our human rights.

Bibliography

All links accessed January–March 2021

6–11
C. Quint, "The Period Positive Pledge", *Disrupted* 4.2, CFFP (2020). *Period Positive*, www.periodpositive. com. C. Quint, *Adventures in Menstruating*, (zine). C. Quint, "From embodied shame to reclaiming the stain", *Soc Rev* 67, no. 4 (2019).

14–17
L. Catalini and J. Fedder, "Characteristics of the endometrium in menstruating species", *Biol Reprod* 102, no. 6 (2020). Pliny the Elder, *The Project Gutenberg EBook of the Natural History of Pliny*, volume 4 (of 6). H. King, "The History of Menstruation", https://www.wondersandmarvels.com/2013/02/ the-history-of-menstruation, 2013. J. Grahn, *Blood, Bread, and Roses*, Beacon Press, 1993. E. Van de Walle and E. Renne (eds), *Regulating Menstruation*, University of Chicago Press, 2001. S. Joseph, *Ṛtu Vidyā*, Notion Press, 2020. R. Paudel, *Dignified Menstruation*, Kathmandu, 2020.

18–19
S. Reid, "Thy Righteousness is but a menstrual clout", *Early Modern Women* 3 (2008). S. Reid, *Maids, Wives, Widows*, Pen and Sword, 2015. L. Smith, "The Shame of Menstruation", *Liberation Collective*, Jul 2013, liberationcollective.wordpress.com. S. Ives, "Tidbits on Mid-Victorian Era Menstrual Hygiene", *Susanna Ives*, Sep 2015, susannaives.com. L. Freidenfelds, *The Modern Period*, Johns Hopkins University Press, 2009.

20–21
L. Bushak, "A Brief History Of The Menstrual Period", *Medical Daily*, May 2016, medicaldaily.com. J. Antonovich, "See Sally Menstruate", *Nursing Clio*, Aug 2012, nursingclio.org. E. Kissling, *Capitalizing on the Curse*, Rienner, 2006. Ad*Access, repository.duke.edu/ dc/adaccess.

24–25
E. Martin, *The Woman in the Body*, Beacon Press, 2001.

B. Fahs, "Demystifying Menstrual Synchrony", *Women's Reprod Health* 3, no. 1 (2016)

26–27
H. Sveen, *Lava or Code Red: A Linguistic Study of Menstrual Expressions in English and Swedish*, www. tandfonline.com, 2016.

32
J.M. Wood, *The Palgrave Handbook of Critical Menstruation, (In)Visible Bleeding: The Menstrual Concealment Imperative*, 2020.

34–35
C. Quint, "I've stopped saying 'feminine hygiene products'", *Independent*, Oct 2017, independent.co.uk.

37–39
R. Steward et al., "'Life is Much More Difficult to Manage During Periods'", *J Autism Dev Dis* 48 (2018). "Sexual assault: ACOG Committee Opinion No. 777", *Obstet Gynecol* 133 (2019). L. Sobel and D. O'Rourke-Suchoff, "Providing Obstetric Care for Women with a History of Sexual Trauma", *HCP Live*, Feb 2019, hcplive.com. "What is PME?", *IAPMD*, Dec 2020, iapmd.org. K. Cathey, "Alphabet Soup Gone Wrong", *PsychCentral*, Jun 2016, psychcentral.com. C. McWeeney, "Menstruating while disabled", *Clue*, Feb 2018, helloclue.com. E. Wright, "Moon Cups Are Not For Me", *Medium*, 2020, medium. com. J. Bell, "What it's like to get your period when you're trans", *Clue*, Feb 2019, helloclue.com. Y. Van Baarsen, "Gender-neutral menstruating", *Period!*, Jun 2020, period.media. L. Ross, "Reproductive Justice as Intersectional Feminist Activism", *Souls* 19, no. 3 (2017). "Reproductive Justice", *Sister Song*, sistersong.net.

40–43
C. Bobel, *The Managed Body*, Palgrave Macmillan, 2018. V. Newton, *Everyday Discourses of Menstruation*, Palgrave Macmillan, 2016. C. Quint, "What if...?", *The Sex Educational Supplement* 2, no. 3 (2016). C. Quint, "Period Positive Menstruation Education Programme of Study", *Period Positive*, 2018, periodpositive.com. S. King, *Menstrual Matters*, menstrual-matters.com. Sheffield Hallam SU, "#PeriodPositive Union", 2018.

46–47
"Vasovagal syncope", *Mayo Clinic*, 2021, mayoclinic.org.

48–49
Anatomy of the clitoris https://onlinelibrary.wiley.com.

51–55
"Heavy periods: overview", *NHS*, Jun 2018, nhs.uk.
A. Marcin, "Black, Brown, Bright Red, and More",
Healthline, Mar 2019, healthline.com.

56–57
C. Quint, "From embodied shame to reclaiming the
stain", *Soc Rev* 67, no. 4 (2019).

58–59
"Cumulative exposure and feminine care products",
Safe Cosmetics, 2018, safecosmetics.org.

62–63
Museum of Menstruation & Women's Health, mum.org

72–73
"Toxic shock syndrome", *NHS*, Sep 2019, nhs.uk.
M. Ellis, "Everything You Need to Know About Vaginal
Discharge", *Healthline*, Nov 2019, healthline.com.

78–79
V. Jain and V. Wotring, "Medically induced amenorrhea
in female astronauts", *npj Microgravity* 2 (2016). L.
Christopher and L. Miller, "Women in War", *Military
Med* 172, no. 1 (2007). *Period and Menstrual Hygiene
Equality Guide*, www.archaeologists.net.

88–89
D. Morris et al., "Familial concordance for age at
menarche", *Paed & Perinatal Epidem* 25, no. 3 (2011).
S. Bradley et al., "Precocious puberty", *Br Med J* 368, no.
6597 (2020). "Early or delayed puberty", *NHS*, Mar 2019,
nhs.uk. J. Millar, "Late period or early miscarriage?",
My Fertility Focus, Augt 2019, myfertilityfocus.com.

94–95
K. Fehlner et al., "The Premenstrual Syndrome and
the Partner Relationship", *J Preg Reprod* 1, (2018).

96–97
M. Hill, *Period Power*, Bloomsbury, 2019. S. Weiss,
"Your Menstrual Cycle Might Be Able to Determine
When to Break Up", *Glamour*, Apr 2017, glamour.com.
A. Laird, *Heavy Flow*, Dundurn, 2019.

98–99
N. Panay, "Guidelines on premenstrual syndrome", *NAPS*,
2018. E. Smith, "Period Poop: It's A Thing", *Refinery29*,

Feb 2020, refinery29.com. "Help! I think I have PMDD!",
Vicious Cycle, viciouscyclepmdd.com. "Bipolar
Disorder and PMDD", *IAPMD*, Nov 2020, iapmd.org.

100–101
M. Deutsch, "Information on Testosterone Hormone
Therapy", *UCSF Transgender Care*, Jul 2020,
transcare.ucsf.edu. S. Frank, "Queering Menstruation",
Sociol Inq 90, no. 2 (2020).

102–103
J. Shaw, "Acne: effect of hormones on pathogenesis
and management", *Am J Clin Dermatol* 3, no. 8 (2002).

106–107
"Guideline on the management of women with
endometriosis", ESHRE, Sep 2013. "Treatment:
Endometriosis", *NHS*, Jan 2019, nhs.uk. "International
evidence-based guideline for the assessment and
management of polycystic ovary syndrome 2018",
Monash University. Verity, verity-pcos.org.uk.

108–109
"Gynaecological cancers", *The Eve Appeal*,
eveappeal.org.uk. www.kff.org/womens-health-
policy/fact-sheet/the-hpv-vaccine-access-and-use-in-
the-u-s. www.womenshealth.gov/a-z-topics/
pap-hpv-tests

112–113
T. Weschler, *Taking Charge of Your Fertility*,
HarperCollins, 2002. "FSRH Clinical Guidance: Fertility
Awareness Methods", Nov 2015. R. Nail, "All About
Conception", *Healthline*, Aug 2018, healthline.com. "Low
sperm count", *Mayo Clinic*, Oct 2020, mayoclinic.org.

114–115
"Should I freeze my eggs? A guide to the latest
information and statistics on egg freezing in the UK",
HFEA, Sep 2018. "Frozen eggs storage 10-year limit
'should be changed'", *BBC*, Oct 2019, bbc.co.uk.

116–117
"Conditions that affect fertility", *Harvard Health
Publishing*, May 2009, health.harvard.edu. T. Weschler,
Taking Charge of Your Fertility, HarperCollins, 2002.
"Infertility", *NICE*, Aug 2018, cks.nice.org.uk.

118–119
"Fertility problems: assessment and treatment", NICE,

Sep 2017, nice.org.uk. A. Rodrigo et al., "Process of IVF with donor sperm", *Invitra*, Oct 2017, invitra.com.

120–125

"Combined pill", NHS, Jul 2020, nhs.uk. "The progesterone-only pill", NHS, Feb 2021, nhs.uk. A. Edelman et al., "Continuous or extended cycle vs. cyclic use of combined hormonal contraceptives", Cochrane Db System Rev no. 7, (2014). C. Read, "New regimens with combined oral contraceptive pills", Eur J Contr Reprod Health Care 15, no. 2 (2010). "What should I do if I miss a pill?", NHS, Feb 2019, nhs.uk. "Your contraception guide", NHS, Mar 2021, nhs.uk. "Intrauterine device" and "Intrauterine system", NHS, Feb 2018, nhs.uk. M. Llamas, "Mirena Insertion", Drugwatch, Mar 2021, drugwatch.com.

126–127

H. Grigg-Spall, *Sweetening the Pill*, John Hunt Publishing, 2013. G. Birnbaum et al., "The Bitter Pill", *Evol Psychol Sci* 5, no. 3 (2019). A. Alvergne and V. Lummaa, "Does the contraceptive pill alter mate choice in humans?", *Trends Ecol Evol* 25, no. 3 (2009).

128–129

"Your contraception guide", *NHS*, Mar 2021, nhs.uk. "FSRH Clinical Guidance: Fertility Awareness Methods", Nov 2015. "Justisse Method", justisse.ca.

132–133

"Symptoms of pregnancy: What happens first", *Mayo Clinic*, May 2019, mayoclinic.org.

134–135

https://www.plannedparenthood.org/learn/morning-after-pill-emergency-contraception/whats-ella-morning-after-pill https://bnf.nice.org.uk/drug/ulipristal-acetate.html#indicationsAndDoses. https://www.plannedparenthood.org/learn/morning-after-pill-emergency-contraception/whats-plan-b-morning-after-pill.

136–137

J. Kline, "Conception to Birth – Epidemiology of Prenatal Development", in *Monographs in Epidemiology and Biostatistics*, Oxford University Press, 1989. Sands, sands.org.uk. https://www.cdc.gov/ncbddd/stillbirth/facts.html.

138–139

C. de Bellefonds, "Postpartum Bleeding (Lochia)", *What to Expect*, Feb 2020, whattoexpect.com.

142–143

M. Guilló-Arakistain, "Challenging menstrual normativity", in C. Bobel et al. (eds), *Palgrave Handbook of Critical Menstruation Studies*, Palgrave Macmillan, 2020.

144–145

L. Foxcroft, *Hot Flushes, Cold Science*, Granta, 2011. M. Perianes and E. Kissling, "Transnational Engagements", in *Palgrave Handbook of Critical Menstruation Studies*, Palgrave Macmillan, 2020. Rock My Menopause, rockmymenopause.com/. "British Menopause Society Fact Sheet: National survey – The results", 2020. Menopause Cafe, menopausecafe.net.

146–147

G. Mansberg, *The M Word*, Allen & Unwin, 2020. "BMS Fact Sheet", 2020. M. Nosek et al., "Effects of Perceived Stress and Attitudes Toward Menopause and Aging...", *J Midwifery Wom Health* 55, no. 4 (2010). G. Jack et al., "Menopause in the workplace", *Maturitas* 85 (2016). https://thebms.org.uk/2016/05/women-suffering-silence-new-bms-survey-puts-spotlight-significant-impact-menopause.

148–149

"Menopause: diagnosis and management, NICE guideline", Dec 2019. "Hormone replacement therapy: overview", *NHS*, Sep 2019, nhs.uk. "Understanding the risks of breast cancer", Women's Health Concern, Mar 2017. R. Crofford, "Differences between compounded BHRT and conventional HRT", *PMFA J* 6, no. 6 (2019).

150–151

"FSRH Guideline: Contraception for Women Aged Over 40 Years", Sep 2019. J. Davis, "Sex drive & menopause", *Rock My Menopause*, 2019, rockmymenopause.com. www.menopausecafe.net. https://www.mayoclinic.org/diseases-conditions/menopause/expert-answers/testosterone-therapy/faq-20057935.

See also: www.dk.com/bpp-biblio

Index

About the author and consultant

Chella Quint is a designer, writer, performer and period educator, originally from Brooklyn, New York, now based in Sheffield. She graduated from NYU Tisch School of Arts then moved to the UK to teach. She became head of her school's PSHE department before becoming one of the UK's top experts on menstruation education. Her solo comedy shows, public engagement projects, design installations, and print zine have inspired and informed adults and children alike in the UK and internationally. Chella founded the Period Positive movement and #periodpositive, an initiative which challenges menstrual taboos and advocates for better menstrual literacy: the cornerstone of any initiative to address period poverty, period equity, education, and menstrual wellbeing. She is currently researching a PhD in design and health.

Dr Shehnaaz Jivraj (medical consultant) is a consultant obstetrician and gynaecologist at the Jessop Wing of Sheffield Teaching Hospitals NHS Trust, and a consultant at Yorkshire Fertility and Menopause Solutions. She is an honorary senior lecturer at the University of Sheffield and a member of the Equality and Diversity Committee of the Royal College of Obstetricians and Gynaecologists.

Acknowledgments

Author acknowledgments

To my family: especially my mom, Annette Quint, for starting me on this journey and always encouraging me. To Laura, Lolo, Shelly, Sharon, Aviva, and the rest of the Quint, Gaber, Gottlieb, Veni and Lauria crews. In memory of Kitty, Harry, Stan, and Sam. For moral support during lockdown, and always: Thomas McCart, Alice Wareham, and Bajsie. Draft readers and cheerleaders: Erin Hawley, Sarah Boyd, Rowena Fletcher-Wood, Angela Brett, Lindsay Keith, Jess Nixon, Juliette Totterdell, Frankie Arundel, SHWI, North American Ladies, Period Positive Award holders and Global Champions. To the SMCR, especially my Period Mom: Chris Bobel, and Period Aunties: Liz Kissling, Laura Wershler, Peggy Stubbs and Breanne Fahs. To Dr Shehnaaz Jivraj for her guidance and humour and her husband Mehmud Nathu for cheering us on over Zoom. To DK: Dawn Henderson, Salima Hirani, Megan Lea, Emma Hill, and Natalie Clay. Finally to the readers, audiences and supporters of Period Positive who weren't afraid to ask questions.

Publisher's acknowledgments

DK would like to thank: Céleste Wallaert for working tirelessly on the illustrations; Kiron Gill for editorial assistance; Kelly Thompson for proofreading; and Ruth Ellis for providing the index.

This book follows the Period Positive Pledge. For more information, visit www.periodpositive.com